PRAISE FOR *NATURE WANTS US TO BE FAT*

"A calorie is NOT a calorie. Dr. Richard Johnson explains how a simple mutation turned a simple sugar, fructose, ostensibly an energy source, into a metabolic poison that foments the chronic diseases that plague America, and indeed the rest of the world."

—Robert Lustig, MD, MSL, UCSF neuroendocrinologist and author of *Metabolical*

"A fascinating look at the science of obesity, with many practical tips. Dr. Johnson points out that 'It is not our culture that is making us fat. It is our biology' and proceeds to explain that biology from an evolutionary viewpoint. An important book."

—Jason Fung, MD, author of the *Obesity Code*

"Rick has spent his career elucidating the unique metabolic properties of fructose in a way that has brought immense clarity to the field. I have learned a great deal from his research, and it has shaped how I think about nutrition science, insulin resistance, NAFLD, type 2 diabetes, and the cluster of metabolic diseases that link to metabolic syndrome. By providing an evolutionary explanation for fructose's unique metabolic role, he takes the emotion out of a very charged topic and lets the biology speak for itself."

—Peter Attia, MD, founder of Early Medical and host of *The Drive* podcast

"This fascinating and provocative book makes the case that fructose has a unique role to play in the development of diabetes, obesity, and other chronic diseases. Is there a 'fat switch' and can we reverse it? Dr. Johnson takes us on an entertaining, wide-ranging journey through animal and human studies as well as stories from the history of humankind, to provide some rigorous answers."

—Nina Teicholz, science journalist and author of the international bestseller author of *The Big Fat Surprise*

"What if fructose is the key common denominator that is making and keeping us fat? Dr. Johnson presents a compelling, meticulously researched case for why nature has exquisitely designed our bodies to store fat in response to excess fructose—and how that knowledge can dig us out of the monumental metabolic disease epidemic we are in. You'll learn not only how fructose is driving our survival mechanism ('the survival switch') to store fat, but also how surprising factors like dehydration, umami flavors, and even low vitamin C contribute directly as well. Metabolic dysfunction is ravaging the globe, with an incalculable toll of lost lives, human suffering, and medical costs. This book is an evidence-based lifeline and a practical path forward for any individual who wants to lose weight, take control of their health, and understand the impact of food on the body."

—Casey Means, MD, metabolic health physician and co-founder of Levels

"Dr. Johnson is a prolific scientist who has made amazing discoveries on the metabolism of fructose and its relation to health. In this latest book, he presents a credible new theory to explain why more and more people are getting fatter and sicker and what can be done about it. This is a rare book that breaks down decades of impactful scientific work into something easily digestible. As such, I consider it highly valuable reading for researchers and health-care professionals, while being easily accessible to the layperson as well."

—Jeff Volek, PhD, RD, professor at the Ohio State University, co-founder and chief science officer at Virta Health, and author of *The Art and Science of Low Carbohydrate Living* and *The Art and Science of Low Carbohydrate Performance*

"Rick Johnson is a top-notch scientist and a gifted writer. He has been at the forefront of research on human nutrition and physiology and has developed a novel understanding to explain at the metabolic level why we are destined to gain weight and what to do about it. In his new book, Rick writes about the latest research on this topic in very approachable and easily understood terms and artfully blends this with real-life examples from nature and cultural references to make for a very compelling, informative, and fun read."

—Michael Goran, MD, author of *Sugarproof*

"Because of my interest in the connection between diet and brain function, I have closely followed the articles and books published by Richard Johnson. He has always been at the leading edge of diet and health issues, especially when it comes to the central role of fructose. His new book, *Nature Wants Us to Be Fat*, sets a new standard when it comes to understanding the pathology of obesity and metabolic disorders. He presents a complete science-based description of the underlying pathology, and he uses this information to give us revolutionary new tools to reverse obesity and metabolic disorders. This book is a 'must read' for the medical and scientific communities, as well as for the general public."

—William L. Wilson, MD, family physician and author of *Brain Drain*

"Despite all the sickening stereotypes about fat people being lazy, stupid, and incapable of controlling their food intake, the reality is that the kind of food we eat matters when it comes to packing on the pounds. By zeroing in first on the fructose aspect of weight gain, Dr. Richard Johnson has been on the cutting edge of this issue for many years. After digging even deeper into this topic, he now realizes that there is more to the obesity story than mere fructose consumption. *Nature Wants Us to Be Fat* gets into the nuts and bolts of exactly how we got here and what it will take to deal with the obesity epidemic once and for all. Fantastic read!"

—Jimmy Moore, international bestselling author of *Keto Clarity*

"With authority and clarity, *Nature Wants Us to Be Fat* presents critical insights into the challenges of obesity. Johnson, an authority in the field, presents a powerful new framework for understanding why we gain weight, why it is so difficult to lose weight, and the most effective strategies for maintaining optimal weight and health. *Nature Wants Us to Be Fat* presents many crucial insights with salience for health professionals, patients, and anyone interested in understanding and effectively approaching challenges of overweight and obesity in their own lives."

—Barbara N. Horowitz, MD, Harvard professor and coauthor of *Zoobiquity*

"Professor Rick Johnson, author of *The Fat Switch*, has written a must-read and delightful follow-up book full of interesting information describing the surprising science behind weight gain. Through an understanding of our ancestral genetics and studies of nature, the author uses a biomimetic approach to explain and understand the power of fat and why obesity has turned out to be a *pandemic in slow-motion*. Read this book and learn from one of the most popular scientific writers why nature wants us to be fat."

—**Peter Stenvinkel, MD, Karolinska Institutet, international expert and advocate for how nature can teach us about medicine**

"*Nature Wants Us to Be Fat* is a book that must be read. It describes the journey of a recognized scientist moving back and forth from observations in zoology and anthropology to rigorous laboratory observations, leading to the conclusion that nature's defense mechanisms are at the root of obesity and other present-day diseases. The journey itself is recounted in a fluid and enthralling way that makes it impossible to put the book to rest until the last page is turned."

—**Bernardo Rodriguez-Iturbe, MD, professor of medicine and past president of the International Society of Nephrology**

"Professor, clinician, obesity researcher, and author, Richard Johnson, MD, in his new book *Nature Wants Us to Be Fat* takes a unique look at the root causes of obesity and chronic disease. From an evolutionary standpoint, he explains how we eat to survive—yet in a modern world full of excess there is a mismatch between our need to eat and our environment filled with refined and processed foods that drive our appetite and make us gain fat. He explains the unique role of fructose and uric acid as triggers to gain fat and drive chronic disease and what we can do to prevent and reverse these conditions. I would highly recommend this well written and easy to understand book to the general public and other health-care professionals."

—**Jeffry N Gerber, MD, FAAFP, Denver's Diet Doctor and co-organizer Low Carb Conferences**

"This is an amazing book and could be described as Johnson's odyssey through the maze of why so many of us are becoming obese and developing type 2 diabetes. He intersperses the book with wonderful examples of other animals that deliberately make themselves fat in order to survive adverse circumstances. This so-called survival switch is, according to Johnson, the secret of why we are all getting fat. Most of us now live in a world of excess whereas we evolved in a world where we had to survive with sudden scarcities of food. Therefore, the survival switch is now harming us.

The narrative of the book is about how fructose turns on the survival switch—making us obese—when we have no need for it. Hypothesis follows hypothesis, with experiments that Johnson himself and his collaborators have largely carried out to prove or disprove the theory.

A very readable and entertaining book."

—**Graham MacGregor, CBE, FRCP, professor of cardiovascular medicine, Wolfson Institute, Chair of Barts and London Hospital Medical school UK, and Chair of Action on Salt and Sugar**

Nature Wants Us to Be Fat

ALSO BY RICHARD J. JOHNSON, MD

The Sugar Fix
The Fat Switch

Nature
Wants Us
to Be Fat

THE SURPRISING SCIENCE BEHIND WHY
WE GAIN WEIGHT AND HOW
WE CAN PREVENT—AND REVERSE—IT

Richard J. Johnson, MD

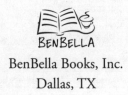

BenBella Books, Inc.
Dallas, TX

Disclosure: Dr. Johnson has received funding from the National Institutes of Health, the Department of Defense, the Veterans Administration, and the State of Colorado. His research and that of his group have led to patents related to fructose and uric acid metabolism. He has equity with XORTX Therapeutics and Colorado Research Partners, LLC, companies making drugs to lower uric acid and block fructose metabolism, respectively. Dr. Johnson has also consulted with Horizon Pharmaceuticals and received honoraria from Danone.

BenBella Books, Inc.
10440 N. Central Expressway
Suite 800
Dallas, TX 75231
benbellabooks.com
Send feedback to feedback@benbellabooks.com

BenBella is a federally registered trademark

Printed in the United States of America
10 9 8 7 6 5 4 3 2 1

Library of Congress Control Number: 2021034768
ISBN 9781637740347 (trade cloth)
ISBN 9781637740354 (ebook)

Editing by Leah Wilson
Copyediting by James Fraleigh
Proofreading by Sarah Vostok and Michael Fedison
Indexing by Amy Murphy
Text design and composition by Aaron Edmiston
Cover design by Faceout Studio, Molly von Borstel
Cover image © Shutterstock / Ralu Cohn
Icon on page 38 by Adrien Coquet, from the Noun Project
Printed by Lake Book Manufacturing

Special discounts for bulk sales are available. Please contact bulkorders@benbellabooks.com.

*To my mentors and role models, including my father, J. Richard Johnson;
William Couser; Seymour Klebanoff; Craig Tisher; Tomas Berl; and
Steven Benner. To my family, Olga, Tracy, and Ricky, and to my patients,
to whom I am grateful for the opportunity to oversee their care.*

Contents

Foreword

Natural selection—or more appropriately, genetic selection—is the process whereby the environment in which a particular organism lives "selects" specific variations in genetic constitution that are most advantageous for survival, and these variations are passed from generation to generation. As such, whether the genetic makeup of an organism proves salubrious or not is very much context dependent, as it relates to the environment in which it is trying to survive.

For the most part, environmental changes affecting life on our planet have been relatively slow. The incremental nature of these shifts in variables like temperature and food availability have therefore played well with the selection of random genetic variations that coded for survival in the face of these new environmental challenges—a dynamic process central to the ongoing refinement of the genome of any living organism.

As Dr. Johnson so eloquently reveals, our distant primate ancestors faced such an environmental challenge many millions of years ago. A cooling planet, over millions of years, with its consequent decline in food availability, presented an environmental pressure favoring genes that could maximize survival. This new genetic constitution was one that provided a survival advantage by allowing our distant forebears the ability to more aggressively make and store fat, a powerfully effective physiological advantage during times of food scarcity.

No doubt, these genetic changes provided advantages even for our more recent human ancestors, whose success at hunting and gathering was not always guaranteed. Indeed, for almost the entire history of human existence, our food security has been tenuous.

But with the development of agriculture some fourteen to seventeen thousand years ago, that situation changed quite suddenly and dramatically. This event, the so-called Agricultural Revolution, confronted human physiology with intense environmental stress of a different sort. Within a few short millennia, calories derived mostly from carbohydrate-rich crops became abundant and ultimately dominated the human diet. The change was so rapid that adaptive genetics couldn't come into play. As such, a threatening environmental/evolutionary mismatch took shape that continues to threaten our health to this very day. Our genetic makeup continues to prepare our bodies for food scarcity, making and storing fat whenever we are exposed to an abundance of carbohydrates, particularly fructose. In essence, we are constantly preparing for a winter that never comes.

The Agricultural Revolution is seen as one of mankind's greatest blessings, and rightfully so. Humanity has taken incredible leaps forward as a consequence of improved food security. But through the lens of challenging the ability of our genome to keep us healthy, as evidenced by the more than 2 billion people on our planet who are overweight or obese, there is reason to challenge the universality of support for this cataclysmic shift in human nutrition. As Yuval Noah Harari wrote in his bestselling book, *Sapiens: A Brief History of Humankind*:

> *This is hard for people in today's prosperous societies to appreciate. Since we enjoy affluence and security, and since our affluence and security are built on foundations laid by the Agricultural Revolution, we assume that the Agricultural Revolution was a wonderful improvement.*

Ours is a thrifty genome, a genome geared at regulating our physiology to maximize our chances of survival when faced with food scarcity—a situation unknown to most people in the developed world. And as Dr. Johnson explains, the consequences of this environmental/evolutionary mismatch may well underpin not just weight gain, but a host of other metabolic maladies including diabetes and hypertension.

In an op-ed published half a century ago in the *Miami Herald,* I explored the health implications of our environmental/evolutionary mismatch and concluded by asking: "But what about the people of today who are stuck with the outdated machinery?" Our "machinery," meaning our physiology, is a manifestation of the information provided by our genes and gifted to us from all who have come before. And truly, human physiology, so well adapted to the environments faced by our ancestors, is less well suited to what we experience in our modern world, especially as it relates to food.

Our mission, if we are to achieve better health, is to bring our environment and our genetics into better alignment. And while we cannot as yet speed the evolutionary process or initiate specific changes in our genome to bring it more in line with the world in which we live, we can absolutely influence the environmental side of this relationship.

In the pages that follow, Dr. Johnson leverages more than two decades of dedicated and detailed research in both animal models and humans to create a program that will ultimately set the stage for a harmonious relationship with your DNA. He reveals how fructose sugar uniquely serves as a critical signaling molecule, alerting the body to prepare for food scarcity by augmenting the creation and storage of fat as a caloric reserve and enhancing insulin resistance, the harbinger of type 2 diabetes. And finally, he provides a deep dive into the fascinating science, almost entirely developed by Dr. Johnson, that highlights the central role of uric acid, the ultimate downstream product of fructose metabolism, in the ever-increasing global issues related to all manner of metabolic diseases.

Understanding how our modern-day choices play upon our ancestral genetics opens the door for implementing lifestyle changes for achieving long-sought-after health goals. And this is truly an empowering gift.

—David Perlmutter, MD, FACN
Hunstville, Ontario, Canada
July 2021

The Birth of an Epidemic

On a rainy morning, the first of May, 1893, President Grover Cleveland opened the Chicago World's Fair to more than 129,000 visitors, concluding his speech by pushing a gold-and-ivory button that lit up the entire six-hundred-acre fairgrounds with new electric lights to replace the old gas lamps. Before the fair ended six months later, 27 million visitors had walked through its gates, making it the greatest fair of the nineteenth century and one of the largest events ever held to date in all human history.

The fair celebrated the four hundredth anniversary of the first voyage to America by Christopher Columbus, and so "The Columbian Exposition" was its official name. And indeed, there was much that celebrated the past. Full-size replicas of the *Niña*, the *Pinta*, and the *Santa María* sat in Lake Michigan near Jackson Park and could be boarded by eager visitors who wanted to see what their voyage to America would have been like. Also next to the Exposition was Buffalo Bill's famous *Wild West* show, which chronicled the adventures of the West with horse shows, "Indian" dancers, sharpshooting by Annie Oakley, and storytelling by Calamity Jane.

Most of the visitors, however, were not so much interested in the past, for the Chicago World's Fair was also about the future, and never in human history had the future been so bright. In addition to electric lights, the telephone was now available; a few months earlier the first phone connection between New

York City and Chicago had been established. The first American automobile company had just opened, selling cars with the new gas-powered engine. Phonographs had recently been invented, and one could visit phonograph parlors to hear recordings of concerts and music.

The fair itself was filled with marvels of the modern era, including the first Ferris wheel and the first electric moving walkway, electric gondolas that transported people across the canals and waterways, and the first electric kitchen, boasting the new electric oven as well as an electric water heater and dishwasher. The fair also featured new sugary treats, like caramel popcorn (later named Cracker Jack) and Wrigley's Juicy Fruit gum, along with newly introduced soft drinks served from soda fountains.

Similar to the fields of technology and industry, medicine was also experiencing a golden age. For hundreds of years the great menace had been infectious diseases, with diphtheria, pneumonia, typhoid fever, and cholera racking up major death tolls. Tuberculosis was especially feared, for it could cause high fevers and the chronic coughing up of blood; often the victim would wither away into a shadow before succumbing. Tuberculosis struck down many famous people, including Andrew Jackson, Frédéric Chopin, John Keats, and Jane Austen. No one was safe.

But medicine was making great advances. Infectious diseases were finally being controlled, both by simple hygienic practices such as handwashing and through the introduction of the first vaccines for diseases such as cholera and rabies. Emil von Behring went a step further by developing the first treatment for common bacterial infections. By immunizing horses, Behring was able to make antitoxins to treat diphtheria, which, he soon demonstrated, could cure children suffering from this horrendous infection. Furthermore, just ten years earlier, a young physician by the name of Robert Koch had left the scientific world speechless when he identified the bacteria that caused tuberculosis. With the discovery of the cause of tuberculosis, surely effective treatments were to come. It was a time for rejoicing: the scourge of infectious disease could be defeated, and there was great hope that soon the days of Camelot would be upon us, with sunny days, rainy nights, and promises of long, safe, and healthy lives. Consistent with the temperament of the time, a physician named Arthur Conan Doyle had just published *The Adventures of Sherlock Holmes*, about how the powers of insight and observation can solve even the most difficult problem or mystery.

Unknown to those living back then, however, the world was about to witness an epidemic of staggering proportions. Not that the malady originated in the 1890s; as we will see, it can be traced back much earlier. However, a tipping point was reached at the end of the nineteenth century, when diseases once considered rare began to increase markedly in the general population. The epidemic was also not just one disease, but a medley of conditions. And it is still raging today across America and the world.

This new epidemic has killed millions of people, on par with historic epidemics such as the Black Plague (which killed 40 million between 1347 and 1350) or the Spanish flu (which killed 45 million, then 5 percent of the world's population, between 1918 and 1920). One difference from these earlier epidemics is that this one is not infectious in the usual sense, for it is not passed from one person to another; it involves no virus, bacteria, or parasite. It does not cause fever or even any type of acute illness, at least in its early stages. Instead of killing in days, weeks,

OBESITY

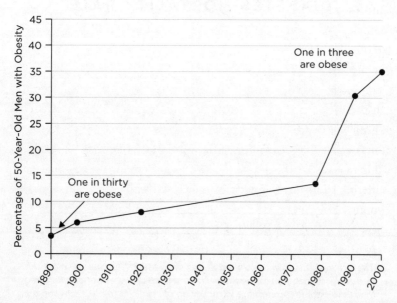

*Obesity has increased dramatically during the twentieth century in the United States. Obesity prevalence (where obesity is defined as a **body mass index**, or BMI, of >30) is shown for fifty-year-old men. (Adapted from Ann Hum Biol 2004; 31174-182.)*

or months, it kills over decades. The epidemic is also so pervasive that physicians today are taught about these conditions as the *normal* diseases of our population. I am talking about not only obesity, but also the diseases that crowd our hospitals today, particularly diabetes, high blood pressure, stroke, and heart disease. Some have referred to these conditions as the *noncommunicable diseases*, and while they may not spread by infection, these diseases are nonetheless now found worldwide, everywhere leaving a swath of morbidity and mortality in their wake.

In 1890, obesity—using the same definition we use today—affected only 3 percent of American adults, and diabetes was present in only two or three out of every one hundred thousand individuals. High blood pressure was seen in fewer than 5 percent of Americans under the age of sixty-five, and coronary artery disease was only being hypothesized as a cause of a rare, strangling chest pain known as angina. Over the last century all this changed.

Today, 30 to 40 percent of the US population is obese, and 10 to 12 percent is diabetic. In some parts of the world, like Samoa, diabetes is present in 40 to 50

DIABETES MORTALITY RATE

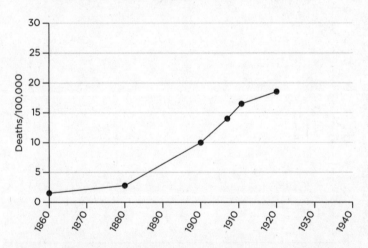

The rise in diabetes in the United States since 1860. This chart displays the frequency of diabetes as the mortality rate from diabetes per one hundred thousand people through the introduction of insulin in the 1920s, when the mortality rate began to fall. (Adapted from Arch Int Med 1924; 34: 585–630.)

percent of the adult population. Likewise, high blood pressure affects one-third of adults, and heart disease is the number one cause of death. Almost no one lacks a family member or friend who suffers from one of these conditions.

The observation that obesity, diabetes, high blood pressure, and coronary artery disease all started to increase sharply beginning in the 1890s raises the question of what common factor might have driven these conditions. What was special about the 1890s that led to the emergence of obesity and these related illnesses? Was it the dramatic improvement in technologies that altered our lifestyle? Was it related to shifting economics, or a specific change in our diet? Later we will return to this time to investigate the primary cause. For now, what most stands out is that neither the public nor physicians were aware of what was around the corner.

Great effort has been devoted to fighting the obesity, diabetes, and heart disease epidemics since the time of that first World's Fair, and enormous progress has been made, at least as it relates to the treatment of diabetes and heart

PREVALENCE OF DIAGNOSED DIABETES IN THE US POPULATION

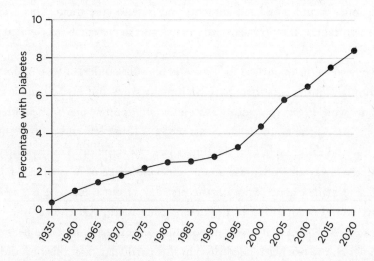

This chart displays the prevalence of diagnosed diabetes as a percentage of the adult population. When undiagnosed diabetes is included, the percentage is higher. For example, in 2020, the total of both diagnosed and undiagnosed diabetes in the US was estimated to be 10.5 percent of the total population, or 13 percent of those eighteen years or older. (Adapted from http://www.cdc.gov/diabetes/data; Am J Pub Health 1946; 36: 26-33.)

disease. We have a library of new treatments for diabetes, including multiple types of insulin and other medications that help control blood glucose levels. We also have an armamentarium of drugs to treat high blood pressure. And if you have heart disease, we have even more options. Anti-smoking campaigns have helped cut heart attacks, and we can lower your cholesterol with medications, inhibit your platelets so your blood is less likely to clot, and even introduce catheters into your heart to open your coronary arteries. It is even possible to replace your heart. The impact of these interventions has been great, and the mortality rates from coronary artery disease in particular have fallen significantly over the last several decades. Yet despite these advances, heart disease remains the number-one killer. And these other epidemics continue to rage.

The problem is that, despite breakthroughs on treatment and management, we still do not have a good understanding of the underlying cause or causes driving these epidemics. Effective treatments are great, but wouldn't it be better if we knew what was causing the problem in the first place? I do not relish the idea of having a catheter put in my heart. Even with great advances in medicine, diabetes disables us, and heart disease hovers like a shadow at the door. We need to know why we are afflicted by these diseases. We need to understand how to prevent obesity and its related ailments and how to cure them. This is all the more important as the prevalence of obesity and diabetes has accelerated since the 1970s.

We need to think outside the box, and consult a different type of doctor.

Throughout the ages there have been many sages, but my favorite is a doctor whose work I read voraciously as a child, and upon whom I can still rely for good advice. As the eminent Dr. Seuss wrote, "Think left and think right and think low and think high. Oh, the thinks you can think up if only you try!"

When I was an undergraduate at the University of Wisconsin, I had a remarkable math teacher who, on the first day of our calculus class, asked us how we would catch a lion in the desert using math. (Of course, one of my classmates responded that it was impossible, since lions do not live in the desert, to which my teacher replied that, in this particular case, this lion did, and it made him all the more hungry.) I thought about this for a few moments, but had no idea what to say. When none of us could answer the question, my teacher explained that the answer was simple. First, you make a fence that crosses through the desert resulting in equal sides. Using binoculars, you then

find out which side the lion is on, and build another fence across that section. You continue to do this until, finally, the lion is contained within a small
fenced-in space. The solution uses the mathematic concept of repeatedly reducing a space by half, an equation in which the answer can never reach zero, but
which will eventually capture any animal with finite size. This was a great lesson
to me: one does not need always to take a standard approach. Taking "the road
less traveled" can be rewarding.

This book presents an unconventional approach followed by myself and
my many collaborators as we have tried to answer the fundamental question
of why we develop obesity and related diseases such as diabetes, heart disease,
high blood pressure, and more. (Our work has found that other diseases not
typically grouped with obesity and diabetes also appear to be related, including
cancer, dementia, and various behavioral disorders.) Our approach is to explore
the question from many angles, including using classical clinical and laboratory studies, as well as lessons from nature, history, and evolution. As a child,
I admired Sherlock Holmes, who could crack impossible cases by the powers
of observation and deduction. Certainly I claim no similarities in talent. Nevertheless, much like the fictional detective's career, mine has led me on many
investigations, where I have needed to ask questions, search for clues, toss aside
false leads, and uncover solid evidence with the hope of getting ever closer to
the truth. My goal was not dissimilar to that presented by my creative math
teacher, but in this case the lion I wished to fence in was the root cause driving
these diseases.

While I am a kidney doctor who continues to see patients, much of my
time is spent doing research. Like most scientists, my research originally was
based on the topic of my specialty. However, each discovery took me down its
own path, in many cases into other fields. My and my team's work expanded
from kidney disease to high blood pressure, diabetes, and even conditions such
as Alzheimer's disease and cancer. I have learned not to be afraid when this happens and—when I step out of my comfort zone—to find experts on that topic
with whom I can collaborate.

When my research took me to the field of obesity, I realized that there was
still so much that was not understood about its underlying cause. If it were
something as simple as eating too much and exercising too little, as had been
touted for decades, then obesity should have been an easy condition to cure.

But then there would not be so many diet plans and exercise routines to choose from, or so much debate as to which approach is best. As it turns out, the problem is not with losing weight itself, because most plans accomplish this. Rather, it is that we rarely sustain our weight loss, as if there is some underlying process that triggers us to regain the fat we fought so hard to lose. Once we are overweight, the excess pounds become an unwelcome companion for years to come.

This made me wonder if there was something missing, some driving cause that still lay hidden, some elusive story that awaited discovery. To find the cause, it seemed, one needed to be resourceful. Although experiments in laboratories or the clinic provide critical insights, by themselves they provide only part of any story. By applying all relevant fields—from classic physiology, genetics, exercise medicine, and nutrition, to fields outside of medicine, including history, evolution, and studies of nature—we gain a fuller picture. As such, our work expanded to include studies of animals in nature (such as hibernating squirrels and bears) and history (from nineteenth-century Europe to the history of Ice Age humans). I am grateful that we have been able to go left, right, high, or low as the clues took us.

In the course of our research, we identified a biological process that animals use to help them survive. This process is most commonly triggered by the food they eat, of which **fructose***—a common type of sugar in our diets—turns out to be especially important, although other foods stimulate it as well. We call it the **survival switch**, as it turns on a whole series of physical and metabolic changes, as well as behaviors, that protect animals in nature when food is not available. One of the features of the switch is that it helps the animal store fat, which can be broken down to provide energy if no food is available. Many humans today have also turned on this switch, and keep it persistently on, with the result that we are now becoming fat. Hence, what was once a survival switch meant to protect us is now a **fat switch** driving obesity. Perhaps more concerning, recent studies suggest that not only is this switch causing obesity and diseases we have long considered related, like diabetes, but that it may have an important role in other conditions, such as heart disease, cancer, and Alzheimer's disease. One of the central discoveries is that obesity is *not the cause of*

---

* Bolded words are defined in the glossary.

these other conditions; rather, obesity and its associated diseases are all driven by the same underlying biological process, the survival switch.

I originally wrote about this switch in 2012 in *The Fat Switch*, but since then we have learned much more about how it works, what turns it on, and most excitingly, how to turn it off. Although fructose present in sugars added to our food and beverages is the main culprit driving this program, we have identified other foods, and other factors, that turn on the survival switch. This research has yielded new insights into preventing and treating these diseases. Some treatments are already commonly used, such as low-carbohydrate diets and intermittent fasting. But we have also found other solutions that are not well known and typically have not been recommended. I am excited to discuss these new approaches with you in this book.

Although our work has not yet been fully accepted by the entire scientific community, this is not uncommon when scientific discoveries are first made. Importantly, our work is based on strong science and has been published in reputable journals, and much of it has been supported by clinical studies.

So let us think outside the box as we attempt to solve the mystery of the greatest epidemic of all time. But where should we begin? Here, we could follow the good Sherlock Holmes advice: "Before we start to investigate, let us try to realize what we do know, so as to make the most of it and to separate the essential from the accidental." Let's start with understanding how obesity can be good. For that, we will want to learn from nature—for it is here that we may find some of the earliest clues to why animals, us included, become fat.

PART I

Why Nature Wants Us to Be Fat

CHAPTER 1

The Power of Fat

Obesity—the condition of having excess fat—is commonly viewed as bad and unhealthy. One reason is that obesity is often accompanied by elevated blood pressure, high concentrations of **triglycerides** (a type of fat in the blood and liver), and high blood sugar levels. These clinical features are consistent with a prediabetic state, and indeed, many individuals with obesity develop diabetes over time. This condition has been given the name **metabolic syndrome**, and is seen as abnormal—as a disease.

In nature, however, obesity is not undesirable. In fact, it is often planned. Obesity is a savior that allows animals to survive deadly winters or droughts and natural disasters. So we have a paradox: fat is bad, but fat is good. How, then, do we understand why fat appears to be a problem for us?

One trick may be to start not with obesity's association with diabetes and heart disease, but with its benefits, and why nature views it differently from how we do. If we understand how fat is beneficial, perhaps we can find out why and how animals trigger their weight gain. This information might then give us our first clues toward solving the riddle of what is causing us to gain weight, why it is associated with poor health, and why that weight is so hard to lose.

Let's begin with one of obesity's champions, the emperor penguin, which I view as the King of Fat.

LEARNING FROM NATURE

Although there was once a penguin, the colossus penguin, that was over six feet tall, today the largest penguins in the world are the emperors, members of a species that lives in Antarctica. Majestic birds that can reach four feet in height, they normally weigh forty to fifty pounds and live along the coast, where they feast on a diet of fish, krill, and squid. They are fast swimmers and great divers, and can submerge for twenty minutes and reach depths of 1,500 feet, making them the deepest-diving birds.

During the Antarctic winter, they nest. A month or two before nesting, the emperors start gaining weight, nearly doubling in size as early winter approaches. They accumulate fat all over their bodies, making some look comically large. The birds then waddle inland at a speed of one to two miles per hour to get away from coastal predators such as leopard seals and killer whales. Twenty-five to forty miles inland, they mate. The mother then lays a single egg and returns to the sea to obtain more food. Meanwhile, the male toughs it out, cradling the egg between his feet and bottom to keep it warm as temperatures fall to −40 degrees Celsius or less. If the winds get fierce, the penguin might huddle with others to protect himself from the cold.

For two months he sits quietly with the egg protected under him, all the time fasting. The large amount of fat he has collected provides both insulation from the freezing temperatures and the calories he needs to live while nesting. The male penguin is larger than the female and can survive longer without food, since he carries more fat. Even then, if his fat stores run out before the egg hatches, he will abandon it and try to get back to the sea in order to find food to survive. Most of the time, however, the male penguin has enough fat, and by the time the chick is born, the mother has returned, often with food that she can regurgitate up for the baby. Then the male can leave to feed and regain his weight.

Other animals put on fat at specific times of the year to help them survive periods when food is scarce. For example, long-distance migrating birds commonly eat more prior to their big flights. These birds become quite fat, which provides the energy they need to make the journey. The European garden warbler will risk crossing the Sahara Desert to its winter habitat in tropical Africa once it has enough fat stores. But the record breaker for distance is the bar-tailed godwit, a seashore bird that uses its long beak to probe sand or mud for insects and crustaceans and builds up fat stores in both its body and liver in late fall before migration. One godwit was documented to have flown seven thousand miles in an eight-day nonstop flight from Alaska to New Zealand.

Animals that **hibernate** also increase their food intake in the fall to build up fat in preparation for the cold winter ahead. To reduce the amount of energy they burn, they slow their metabolism, the chemical reactions that support life. By eating more while using less energy, more of the food these animals eat is turned into fat. Then, when the animals hibernate, they drop their body temperature to near freezing to slow their heart rate and metabolism even more, so that they almost seem dead.

At the university where I work, we have a hibernaculum, a temperature- and light-controlled room that allows us to study the behavior of animals in winter, including that of the thirteen-lined ground squirrel. When these animals hibernate, they will drop their body temperatures to 4 degrees Celsius. Even though they seem almost like rocks when you pick them up, they are not lifeless; their hearts are pumping, they are breathing ever so slowly, and they are slowly burning their excess fat to provide them with the energy they need to survive the long winter months.

In the Amazon lives the pacu fish, which looks like a giant piranha without the sharp teeth. It is a vegetarian, and its favorite food is fruit. Each year, the pacu wait until the heavy rains flood the Amazon; the river rises thirty to forty feet, and spreads into the jungle for miles, deluging as much as 27,000 square miles of forest. Many fruit trees ripen during this flood and drop fruit into the river. The pacu loves the fruit and eats so much that it triples its fat content. Then the flood recedes, the Amazon once again becomes a river, and the fruit is no longer available. The pacu lives for up to six months without food, surviving off its fat, until the Amazon floods again and the fruit is available once more.

As you can see, fat is not a bad thing, if you live in the wild. Sure, you do not want to have so much fat that it slows you down while you are escaping a predator, but it provides a key protection when food is unavailable. In this case, it may be worth rethinking nature's law: it may not always be the fittest that survive. In some situations, it may be the fattest.

Fat is not a bad thing, if you live in the wild.

We usually think of obesity in humans as a disadvantage. But perhaps we have not considered it from nature's perspective. Let us revisit obesity in humans, in light of this paradox, beginning with a tale of two fasts.

A TALE OF TWO FASTS

For over twenty years, a humble lawyer by the name of Mahatma Gandhi led campaigns for the independence of India from the British Empire. He would dress in a loincloth traditionally worn by the poor, and only ate vegetables because he did not believe in killing animals for food. He would protest by walking in long marches; it has been calculated that he walked an average of ten miles a day during this twenty-year period, or the equivalent of walking around the Earth twice. One of his most effective ways of protesting was threatening to fast to his own death, and he did this seventeen times; his longest fast was twenty-one days. In a world where protesting is so commonly violent, the conviction of a humble man to fast himself to death as an act of nonviolent resistance had a major impact. In part because of his leadership and action, India received its independence from England on August 15, 1947.

Independence, however, was not the end of Gandhi's work. India was home to several different religious groups, including Hindus, Muslims, and Sikhs, between which there was friction. As part of the Indian Independence Act, England separated India into two countries, India and Pakistan, with India meant for the Hindus and Pakistan for the Muslims.

Unfortunately, establishing countries by religion placed the religious minorities living in these countries in a difficult situation, and shortly after the establishment of independence there were local uprisings and riots. Hindus and Sikhs were massacred in Pakistan, and Muslims were killed in Calcutta and Delhi. Gandhi called for moral responsibility, asking the government as well as religious groups to stop the fighting and to protect religious minorities in both countries. Unfortunately, the death toll continued to rise.

Finally, in January 1948, Gandhi announced he would fast to his death or until "peace is restored to Delhi and a Muslim can walk around in the city all by himself." After a meal of goat's milk, vegetables, and fruit juice, he began his fast in New Delhi. He was now seventy-seven years old and his 5-foot, 5-inch frame weighed only about a hundred pounds. Gaunt and determined, with a shawl wrapped around his frail body, he emerged from his room each night to pray and to speak to the crowds, his voice low and almost inaudible. By the third day he was visibly much weaker. An American reporter who visited him while he was sleeping on his cot noted that his face showed signs of suffering. By day five his doctors were gravely concerned for his health, but Gandhi's willpower remained strong. The people of Delhi, as well as people throughout the world, were shaken by this man who would starve himself to death to uphold his beliefs. On the sixth day, leaders from the Hindu, Muslim, and Sikh communities gathered with government leaders and signed a pledge to abide by Gandhi's demand, and Gandhi, weak but triumphant, ended his fast.

Seventeen years later and thousands of miles away, a twenty-seven-year-old man by the name of Angus Barbieri checked in at a hospital in Dundee, Scotland, to lose weight. For several years, he had worked in a fish-and-chips shop owned by his father and had progressively gained weight, reaching just over 450 pounds on the day of admission. He was interested in a relatively new approach that was being used to treat obesity, which was to fast for several weeks. Previous individuals had even fasted for as long as one hundred days, according to a paper published in the *Journal of the American Medical Association* the previous year.

Angus was allowed tea, coffee, and water along with vitamins, but was restricted from eating or drinking anything with calories. Although the initial plan was to fast for "only" a few weeks, he did so well that the fast was continued, month after month, until he had passed more than a year without having any food. Amazingly, he did this without developing any symptoms. During this time, he lost 275 pounds—so much weight that his original pants could now hold three individuals of his newly attained size. Triumphant, he broke the fast with a single boiled egg and some bread and butter. Over the following years he was able to maintain a weight less than 200 pounds, and he went on to live twenty-five more years and raise a family.

Both of these tales together tell an important story about survival and the power of fat. When we do not eat, we have to rely on the food we store in our tissues: our fat, primarily, though some energy is provided by the carbohydrates we store in our liver, muscles, and other tissues, called **glycogen**. Gandhi had almost no fat, so fasting for five days almost killed him, whereas Angus was able to fast for 382 days as an outpatient without a problem. Ironically, one of the reasons Gandhi could be so persuasive politically was that he had minimal fat stores—if he had been fat, the impact of his fasting would have been lost.

The take-home message is that fat provides the fuel we need to survive when food is not available. The more fat we have, the longer we can fast. Of course, for Gandhi and Angus, fasting was voluntary.* But what if there is no choice?

AN ADVANTAGE TO BEING MILDLY OVERWEIGHT

When I was working at the University of Washington Hospital in Seattle, I would go two or three times a week to exercise at the university gymnasium across the street. Although I was never a great athlete, I would spend thirty to forty-five minutes lifting weights. Often I would see a friend who was a bodybuilder. He was an incredibly muscular and fit individual, and had absolutely no visible fat. He was ten or even fifteen years older than I but looked ten years younger. He was my role model for what I wanted to look like, and seeing him inspired me to go to the gym even more.

Then, one day, he wasn't there, and I was told he'd been hospitalized for pneumonia. I went to the hospital to find him. When I saw him, I was horrified to see that much of his muscle had disappeared in a matter of days. He looked older and even a bit weak, but his smile was still the same, and I left with feelings of hope. Over the next few days he made a full recovery, and eventually he was able to regain his strength, but it took weeks and weeks.

His problem was that he was all muscle and no fat. This of course made him look fantastic in the gym, but it was not ideal when he got sick. When he developed pneumonia, he lost his appetite and ate minimally, despite needing energy to endure the fever and fight the infection. With no food coming in, and no fat to burn, his body broke down muscle to provide him with the energy he needed. As the muscle melted away, he suddenly looked like he was dying—for when the muscles break down, other systems start to fail, including the liver

---

* If you would like to fast as a means for decreasing your body weight, please read the pros and cons of intermittent fasting versus prolonged fasting in chapter ten first.

and the kidneys. All hell breaks loose. Ironically, if my friend hadn't been so fit—if he'd had some fat to burn instead—his muscle would have been spared and he would not have gotten so sick.

Being mildly overweight is associated with improved survival for people at risk for severe illness, and for individuals more than seventy years old.

Many studies have looked at the ideal weight or amount of fat a person requires to live longer. Given what we've learned, it should not surprise you that being mildly overweight (a BMI of 27)* is associated with improved survival for people at risk for severe illness, such as cancer, heart disease, or kidney failure, and for individuals more than seventy years old. Some studies even suggest that being mildly overweight may be associated with longer life in the general population.

But then how do we explain all the studies that conclude that caloric restriction is associated with living longer? In most laboratory studies that have investigated the effects of caloric restriction, the animals are given about 70 percent of the calories they would normally eat and end up having very little fat, yet live longer than both regular mice and fat mice. Some studies suggest they also age slower than regular mice.

There is also some evidence that this may carry over to humans. The island of Okinawa is famous for having the most centenarians (that is, people who are one hundred years old or older) in the world, and a study of food intake in schoolchildren had suggested that Okinawans may eat approximately one-third less food than Japanese living in other parts of the country. Further support that local dietary habits may be responsible for Okinawans' increased longevity is provided by the finding that individuals who move to other areas of Japan end up having similar life spans as their new neighbors.

I believe the reason that animals on a low-calorie diet live longer is that there is a cost to putting on fat. The food we eat is either broken down into immediate energy (which we call **adenosine triphosphate**, or **ATP**) or turned into stored energy (such as fat). Usually the **calories** we eat are turned into

---

* A BMI of 20 to 25 is considered to be in the normal range, with a BMI of 25 to 30 defined as overweight, and greater than 30 as obese.

immediately available ATP. To instead store these calories for later, our cells must reduce the production of ATP and divert the excess calories to fat. Our research group determined that this is done through exposing the cells' "energy factories" (also known as **mitochondria**), where most of the ATP is produced, to a phenomenon called **oxidative stress**. Thus, the cost of storing fat is some oxidative stress to our energy factories. If sustained for decades, this stress can lead to reduced function in—and even the loss of—these factories, which are responsible for the energy we need to maintain our bodies at full throttle.

So what is oxidative stress? Whenever our body uses oxygen, some of it can be converted into toxic oxygen-containing chemicals that can damage tissues.* Low-grade oxidative stress over time (such as from storing a lot of fat long term) is thought to be the underlying cause of aging, partly due to recurrent damage to our energy factories, which ages us faster. This is why reducing caloric intake can make you both look younger and live longer.

There is a catch, however. Yes, animals that are placed on a low-calorie diet live longer. This is especially true for animals in laboratories, because every day the animals are assured their food intake. However, if these animals were let out in the wild, their survival would be at risk: they have no fat stores, and therefore no protection should there be an unanticipated food shortage, such as from flooding or drought, snowstorm or fire. It would not take much for them to get into trouble.

What about us? Does it make sense to minimize our food stores so we can preserve our energy factories? It may make sense for many of us, as there are a lot of safeguards to protect us against starvation. The average grocery store has over forty thousand different food items. Hospitals have many ways to provide nutrition to sick patients. Nevertheless, an illness can strike so fast that you do not have time to respond, such as what happened with my bodybuilder friend.

In addition, numerous people today lack consistent access to food, whether for economic or other reasons. One estimate suggests that one in nine people in the world experience persistent hunger. Famines, for example, are especially common in African countries such as Ethiopia and Sudan. Most famines are caused by drought, but some are due to war (during which food supplies are

---

* Oxidative stress can also result from things like ultraviolet light, which causes sunburn, and smoking, which may have a role in causing wrinkles.

cut off), crop failures from disease or flood, and other causes. In 1950, a famine occurred in Canada when caribou migration changed, causing starvation among the Inuit, for whom caribou was their main food source. Famines can result in heavy death tolls. The Bengal famine of 1943 resulted in more than 2 million deaths.

Given these considerations, there is not an ideal percentage of body fat that a person should have, as the optimal amount relates to the situation you are in. If you are skinny and keeping your caloric intake low in a society in which food is plentiful, you will likely do well and live long. However, if you have a chronic illness or are older, or if you do not always have good access to food, or if you are in a region at risk for famine, then it is better to have some extra fat on board.

Up to now, we have discussed how fat can aid an individual's survival. However, fat also plays a role in the survival of a species. To survive, the ability of a species to reproduce is paramount, and there is perhaps no other situation where having sufficient fat stores is more important.

PREGNANCY AND THE IMPORTANCE OF BEING SUFFICIENTLY FAT

In pregnancy, it is critical that the mother have sufficient nutrients to provide for her developing baby, and when breastfeeding following birth. This is one reason women of normal weight have evolved to generally carry more fat (25 percent of body weight, on average) than men (who average 15 percent). Rose Frisch, a well-known biologist, determined that women need at least 22 percent body fat to carry a baby to term. According to Frisch, in the absence of food, a pregnant woman would need thirty-five pounds of extra fat to provide enough calories to carry the baby to term and breastfeed for three months.

In our society, most women have plentiful access to food, such that starvation of the baby during pregnancy is not a concern. However, we have medical records from modern famines that allow us to evaluate their impact on pregnant women and their babies. One example is the Dutch famine of 1944–45 during World War II. Netherlands had fallen to Germany in 1940, but by the summer of 1944, much of the southern Netherlands had been freed by the Allies. That September, with Germany slowly weakening, the fugitive Dutch leaders living in

London called for a national railway strike to slow the Nazis. The Nazis retaliated by blocking the delivery of food and fuel to the occupied western Netherlands, including cities such as Amsterdam. This, coupled with a harsh winter, placed 4.5 million people in danger of starving. For six or seven months there was only limited food available, and it had to be rationed. Initially each person was provided 1,000 calories per day (about one-half of normal intake), but as the famine worsened, the number was reduced to 500. In a rare kind gesture, Germany allowed the Royal Air Force, Canadian Air Force, and US Army Air Forces to bring supplies to the starving people in April and May 1945. At least 11,000 tons of supplies were dropped, primarily canned or dried foods and chocolate. But even with these measures, approximately twenty thousand people died.

The effect of the famine on successful pregnancies was substantial. By the peak of the famine, the birth rate had fallen by two-thirds. Those women who did have a successful delivery had less weight gain during pregnancy compared to women in prior years, and those who gained the least, or even lost weight, ended up with smaller-than-normal babies. Very small babies can have a lot of immediate and delayed health issues that affect their development, and may even increase their risk for obesity and high blood pressure as adults. During the famine, conception rates also plummeted, as reflected in the birth rate nine months later. Once a woman's body fat falls below 15 percent, her ovaries' ability to release eggs decreases and menstruation may stop; arrested menstruation and ovulation have also been observed in women with anorexia, ballet dancers, and marathon runners. Starvation also reduces sperm production in men.

While extra body fat may not be so critical for survival in modern society, it was very important in our past. Certainly, it was important during famines. Most famines last months or a few years. However, in 2200 BC (or about 4,200 years ago) there was a drought that lasted a century, one so severe that it is thought to have had an important role in the collapse of the Old Kingdom in Egypt and the Akkadian Empire in Mesopotamia.

While extra body fat may not be so critical for survival in modern society, it was very important in our past.

There was another period of food shortage at the dawn of human history that may not have been as severe, but still set a record, as it lasted more than ten thousand years. The art at that time often consisted of figurines of what appear to be overweight and/or pregnant women. What secrets can we learn from this prehistoric time?

MYSTERIOUS ICE AGE FIGURINES OF OVERWEIGHT WOMEN

The first *Homo sapiens* left Africa about 75,000 years ago, and by 45,000 years ago had arrived in Europe. It was the time of the Last Ice Age, and humans arrived during a brief warm period. These early humans hunted in small bands, bringing down big game such as mammoths, horse, and reindeer that roamed the open grasslands and the tundra that ran along the glacial front. They were sophisticated hunters, with spears made of bone and flint, but their success was soon challenged by a changing climate. About 38,000 years ago, the glaciers once again advanced, bringing colder weather that could reach –10 to –15 degrees Celsius in the winter. Large game decreased in numbers, possibly from overhunting. Soon these early humans began to starve; some groups went extinct, while others migrated south to sheltered, forested valleys where small game was still available. It has been estimated that over a four-thousand- to eight-thousand-year period, the population fell by two-thirds, and the average stature of those who survived decreased by three to four inches.

It was also at this time that the first human art emerged, with beautiful cave paintings of large game animals. Whereas human images are rare in cave paintings, small human figures were frequent subjects of the first sculptures, which were made of mammoth ivory, stone, or (rarely) clay, and were often small enough that they could be held in the hand or worn on a string around the neck. Many have a shiny surface, suggesting that they were handled and probably passed down over the generations.

Most of the sculpted figurines are of naked, overweight women—on the surface a peculiar choice, given they were made at a time when the people were starving. Some also appear to be pregnant. This led some archaeologists to interpret the figurines as signs of beauty, or of fertility, for which reason they were given the name "Venus figurines." Today, however, the term "Venus" is largely considered pejorative, and as such I will refer to them simply as female figurines.

I wondered if these figurines could have represented a symbol of survival for the tribe, or an ideal for women who would have to carry a baby during a brutal period when food might not be available for months. To investigate this possibility, I had the good fortune to work with John W. Fox, a retired professor of anthropology and archaeology from the American University of Sharjah in the United Arab Emirates, and my longtime collaborator, molecular biologist Miguel Lanaspa. We decided that if the hypothesis were true, these figurines would tend to be fatter if made when the glaciers were advancing and climate was cooling, and leaner if made later, when the glaciers receded with the warming climate. We also reasoned that those figurines found closest to the glaciers would be fatter than those found farther away.

To test this idea, we measured the waist-to-shoulder and waist-to-hip ratios of more than forty female figurines. The data supported our hypothesis: figurines made during the glacial advance show greater obesity than figurines from the time of glacial retreat. Furthermore, figurines from the time of the glacial advance were fatter the closer they were to the glacial front.

While most figurines we have that date from this period are female, some male figurines have also been found. These are mostly lean and some have catlike features. Large cats were the greatest predators of the Ice Age. It seems possible that the male figurines represented symbols of the hunt—suggesting the female figurines similarly might symbolize survival of the tribe through successful motherhood.

The idea of obesity as advantageous because it increases the likelihood of a successful pregnancy when food is less available may have passed into modern times. The British adventurer John Speke noted in his travels up the Nile in the 1850s that the royal wives of the king of Karague near Lake Victoria were encouraged to gain fat by being confined to rooms with continuous access to pots of milk and plantains. William Wadd noted similar practices for newlyweds in eighteenth-century Tunisia.

Being modestly obese also could have become viewed as attractive due to its association with fertility and successful pregnancy, much as rosy cheeks are considered attractive because they communicate good health; the women depicted by the figurines could simply have been viewed as beautiful. Peter Paul Rubens, the Flemish artist, is especially famous for his paintings of voluptuous women, which possess an irresistible aura of beauty and charm. Rubens lived in Antwerp in the first half of the seventeenth century, during which time he saw famines, starvation, and plague—of which his first wife died in 1626. But he was also witness to the increasing frequency of obesity among royalty and the wealthy in Amsterdam during that time. I wonder if the contrast of starvation with obesity created greater emphasis on weight as the difference between being sick or healthy, and influenced his impression of how beauty should be viewed.

In sum, carrying fat is not just important for animals in the wild. Early humans recognized that having sufficient fat was critical not just for survival of the individual but of our species. The role of fat in survival also may have had a role in the birth of art and our perception of attractiveness.

Nature wants us to have sufficient fat to survive when situations are rough. To nature, obesity is not unnatural; it is not a disease. Fat is powerful, beneficial, and beautiful—at least in the right setting.

CHAPTER 2

Secret Reasons It Helps to Be Fat

We now have our first clue to the cause of obesity: fat has a purpose. Fat provides calories to animals when they cannot find food. It is a safeguard during times of trouble, and can be critical for survival. Fat is a good guy in nature and, when present, is generally desirable. In our past, we appreciated the power of fat. Today, we have forgotten its importance. We need to change our thinking about fat, from a worthless layer of tissues that weigh on our body to a tool meant to help us when food is not available.

Before we can use this information to figure out what causes obesity, however, we must—as Sherlock would tell us—better understand the scene of the crime. If the production of fat is meant to aid survival, then the scene of the crime is when an animal is preparing for a coming crisis. Fat provides a way to store calories when food is not available, but there are certainly other things that an animal needs to survive. One of the most important is water.

WATER, AN OFTEN
UNAPPRECIATED RESOURCE

When it comes to survival, having adequate fat to provide needed calories is only part of the story. Animals also must have sufficient water. So how do animals get water when it is not available? How does the lungfish get water while burrowed for a year or more under a dried-out lake? How does the hibernating bear get water while in its den for months in the winter cold? How does the bar-tailed godwit get water while flying thousands of miles nonstop over the ocean? Could the way animals survive water shortage have any connection with the way they survive food shortage?

We often take water for granted. Our underappreciation of water is best revealed by a story I first heard in college, about a tribal chief from the jungles of the Amazon who was brought to New York City in the 1930s. As someone experiencing Western civilization for the first time, he must have been amazed to see automobiles and subways, radio and telephones, electricity and lights, tall bridges and towering skyscrapers. After spending a few days seeing all these magnificent inventions, a reporter asked him: What was the most remarkable thing he'd seen? The tribal chief's answer surprised everyone. He thought the most significant invention of the Western world was the simple water faucet.

Cars, elevators, phones, and lights bring comfort and convenience that make life easier. However, for those who live day to day in the jungle with no assurance of what lies ahead, there is nothing more valuable than water. It's no wonder the ability to get water instantly, simply by turning the handle of a faucet, seemed the most miraculous to the tribal chief. Having water translates into survival, and this trumps all other desires.

Today, water shortage is common, affecting approximately one-third to one-half of the world population, especially in South Asia, North Africa, and the Middle East. Some areas have so little water that they are almost uninhabitable. Lack of water is a reason for human migrations and for conflicts leading to war. Water shortages are expected to worsen over the next decades due to expanding populations, pollution, and climate change, so water is once again being recognized as one of our most valuable resources.

SURVIVING WITHOUT WATER IN THE WILD

If humans, with all their technology, cannot depend on having enough water, what about the animals living in the wild? How do animals survive in the desert where water is only rarely available? What happens when there are droughts and no rain for weeks? They can't very well stock up on and carry water bottles, the way we might. With climate change, the world is heating up, and there are more heat waves. Even though average temperatures have increased only 1° Celsius in the last fifty years, the number of extremely hot days has increased markedly. Some studies suggest that three out of every four recent heat waves are caused by climate change. And when temperatures soar, getting dehydrated becomes easy. So how do animals survive?

Many animals have evolved ingenious ways to survive when water supplies dry up. Sure, some animals rely on finding rare water holes and springs, but others have incorporated clever ways to hold on to water. For example, there is a frog that lives in the deserts of Australia that can survive up to five years without water! Perhaps not surprisingly, its name is the water-holding frog, and it stores water in its bladder—sort of like having its own canteen. When a heat spell hits the Great Sandy Desert and causes the few water holes there to dry up, the frog protects itself by burrowing into the ground. Here it lies, in a dormant state similar to a hibernating animal, surviving for months or even years until the rain returns. During this time, it lives off the fat it has previously stored in its feet (where the fat also acted as insulation from the hot sands), and slowly reabsorbs the water that it needs from its bladder. These frogs are so good at storing water that Australia's Tiwi islanders use these frogs as a water source when the water holes have gone dry. They dig the frogs up, then drink the water that the frogs release when they squeeze them over their mouths.*

Turtles and tortoises also store water in their bladders, something that is especially helpful for the tortoises that live in the Galápagos Islands off Ecuador's coast. These volcanic islands have minimal fresh water, as there are no

---

* The importance of these frogs as a water source is clear from the Tiwi myth of Tiddalak, a frog that drank all of the water from the ponds and water holes, leaving nothing for the others, until a wise old owl and a snake got him to laugh so hard that the water came rushing out of his mouth for all to share.

freshwater springs. The only source of water is from the rains, which only amounts to about ten inches per year. The tortoises get their water from cacti and other plants they eat, and by licking dew from rocks in the morning. When the rain comes, they congregate in old water holes and mud holes, where they drink as much water as they can. Then, instead of urinating, the tortoises hold the water in their bladders for months at a time. When the tortoises need water, if they cannot get enough from the food they eat, their bladders then become permeable, allowing the water to be reabsorbed.

Many Galápagos tortoises are huge; they can reach six feet in length and weigh more than eight hundred pounds, and their bladders can store gallons of water. For early sailors who arrived on the Galápagos—and for Charles Darwin and the crew of the HMS *Beagle*—the tortoises were a key source for obtaining water. (They became a favorite food, too, due to their high fat content.)

WHAT ANIMALS DO IF THEY CANNOT STORE WATER

Most animals cannot use their bladders as water bottles, so they need other ways to hold on to water. One way is to reduce the amount of water lost from their bodies through urination. To do this, animals concentrate their urine, giving it lower volume but a deep yellow color and pungent smell. Desert mice have perfected this method, and can concentrate their urine to six times the concentration of seawater.

Another way to hold on to more water is to reduce water loss through the skin, such as from sweating. However, this means forgoing the main benefit of sweating: helping to cool the body. Desert-dwelling camels have fewer sweat glands than most other mammals, so they sweat less and therefore lose less water, but as a consequence, their body temperature rises during the day. (Camels tolerate these higher body temperatures, which in humans would make us feel sick with fever.) Other desert animals instead minimize sweating by hiding in their burrows during the hottest time of the day, and only venture out at night when it is cooler.

All these techniques help reduce water loss from the body. Nevertheless, some loss still occurs, so animals eventually need to replace what is lost. Some supply of water is necessary for survival. So how does the camel, for example, live in the desert for days and weeks without water?

As a kid, I thought that the hump of the camel contained water. I remember being told that it was fat and wondering why a camel would want a pad of fat on the top of its back. The answer might surprise you, because I was sort of right in the first place. The fat in the camel's hump is there to *make* water. When fat is broken down, it provides not only the energy we need to survive, but also water. This is not because there is water *in* fat, but rather because burning fat generates water as one of its by-products.

Accordingly, the state of a camel's hump not only tells you how much fat it's carrying, but also provides a clue as to its water reserves. When the hump is floppy, it is time to get the camel to a natural or artificial spring! This is true for evaluating the body fat in other animals, as well: if an animal appears lean and starving, it could be a sign not only that it needs food, but that it has not been able to find enough water, and had to burn fat to compensate.

The observation that fat is a source of **metabolic water** is rarely discussed in the medical literature, and certainly has been ignored by most investigators studying obesity. It is important to us, however, because it is additional evidence that fat plays a critical role in survival.

FAT AS A SOURCE OF WATER
FOR DEHYDRATED ANIMALS

Naturalists have known for a long time that many animals living in the desert rely on their fat stores to provide metabolic water in times of need. This is a somewhat tricky task, since fat provides insulation that might raise body temperature. To prevent this, many desert mammals, including the kangaroo rat and the jerboa, carry most of their fat in their tails. This is also the reason the camel's fat is stored on a hump on its back, where it does not increase the camel's core temperature the way it would were it spread all over the body.

The need for metabolic water is also a reason marine mammals are commonly fat. The whale is the fattest animal in the world, and while some of the fat serves as insulation in the cold ocean environment, it is also a major source of water. This is because whales, dolphins, and seals do not drink seawater. They get some

Fat is not only a source of calories, but also a source of water.

fresh water from the fish and invertebrates (such as krill) that they eat, and some whales may get a little water by eating ice, but up to one-third of their water comes from burning fat.

It seems that whenever animals have evolved in an environment where water is not readily available, they respond by carrying extra fat. This is similar to animals putting on fat when they know they will have to weather periods in which food is not available. Animals that live where water is scarce must have some extra fat stores all the time. By carrying this fat, they protect themselves in case the water hole or spring goes dry. This is why the Galápagos tortoises are so fat; fresh water is always scarce in the Galápagos Islands, and the fat the tortoises carry provides a critical source of water if rains fail to come. Even desert ants have much bigger fat stores (which are located in "fat bodies") than ants living in temperate or tropical regions, in order to provide water in times of need.

Nature carries many secrets. And if nature designed a process such as gaining fat to help us survive, might not this be coordinated with other biologic changes that could also aid survival? Is it possible that gaining fat is just one part of an orchestrated survival response? If we can better define what comprises this survival response, could it help us identify the cause of obesity? What additional secrets is nature hiding?

Such a survival response, one imagines, would require not only the ability to survive food and water shortages, but also the ability to search effectively for food, defend oneself from predators, and think clearly and make decisions quickly under stress. You would want to conserve as much energy as possible, so as not to burn through your fat reserves before you can access food again. But how does your body do this when you also have to search for that food, while still ensuring your brain is getting enough nutrients to help you out of any desperate situations?

A METABOLIC SURVIVAL RESPONSE

Storing fat is only one approach to an anticipated food shortage; another is to reduce the energy you use. Starving animals, for example, reduce how much energy they use while they are resting, to compensate for energy used while foraging, so that overall they burn less energy than an animal that is not starving. Starving animals are not the only ones that reduce energy use while resting: hibernating animals decrease the amount of energy they use even before they begin hibernation. To survive, in other words, animals do not simply put on fat; they also slow their metabolism so that they are able to keep more of the fat they have stored. As a consequence, they need less energy to keep the body and all its organs functioning. It is as if these animals go into a low-power mode.

However, one organ that nobody wants to short-change is the brain. Survival requires thinking, and thinking requires fuel. Humans, for example, use one-sixth of the calories they ingest just for the brain. When food supplies are low, you want to make sure your brain gets relatively more of the available calories, so it has enough energy to stay fully functional. The body does this by becoming prediabetic. This may sound counterintuitive, as prediabetes is a condition that can progress to diabetes, which is no healthier for other animals than it is for us. However, in situations where survival is key, being prediabetic turns out to be lifesaving.

The brain has a preferred fuel, **glucose**. Normally, glucose is carried in the blood (where it is often referred to as "blood sugar"), from which it is taken up into muscle, the liver, and the brain as a fuel. For glucose to enter muscle and the liver, the hormone **insulin** is required, whereas it can enter most regions of the brain even when insulin is absent. The clever way animals respond to food shortage is by making insulin less effective at moving glucose into muscle and the liver. With less glucose going into these tissues, levels in the blood rise, thereby ensuring sufficient glucose for the brain. This phenomenon is called **insulin resistance**.

Insulin resistance is a major survival response in animals that lack food or water. The hibernating grizzly bear, for example, is insulin resistant during hibernation, allowing its brain to function well even as the rest of its body is living on very little energy. This is why you do not want to wake a bear up by going into its den! Most animals that put on a lot of fat in the wild also become temporarily insulin resistant, including birds that have to fly long distances.

Another part of this survival response is where animals store this extra fat. Fat is normally stored in the **adipose** tissues (the medical term for body fat), which is found in various places in an animal's body, including the abdomen, back, or tail, depending on species. Animals also store fat in the liver and the blood (as triglycerides and cholesterol).

So we see that animals that become obese in nature activate a series of survival responses that include foraging for food, lowering their metabolism, becoming insulin resistant, and increasing fat storage not only in adipose tissues, but also in the liver and blood. This constellation of findings has been observed over and over in hibernating animals including bears, squirrels, and marmots, as well as birds preparing for long-distance travel, and clearly contributes to their survival during periods of food shortage.

A similar constellation of signs is observed in *people* who are overweight or obese, referred to as **metabolic syndrome**. Metabolic syndrome usually refers most specifically to obesity that is most prominent around the abdomen (called "central obesity") in combination with insulin resistance. It is frequently accompanied by increased triglycerides in the blood, as well as a reduction in "good" cholesterol (HDL cholesterol)* and mild elevations in blood pressure. Fatty liver is also common. Today, one-fourth of adults have metabolic syndrome.

For animals in the wild, as hibernation or migration ends, metabolic syndrome has resolved; the extra fat is burned off, and the animal returns to its normal state. For humans, however, metabolic syndrome tends to progress over time. Insulin resistance worsens until glucose levels become persistently high, heralding the onset of diabetes. Blood pressure increases to levels that define it as hypertension, the primary risk factor for stroke and heart failure. The liver keeps accumulating fat while developing inflammation that eventually causes cirrhosis and destroys the organ's tissue. Even the kidneys start losing function over time.

In nature, metabolic syndrome is an insurance plan. For humans today, metabolic syndrome is a disorder, a harbinger presaging the development of diabetes, high blood pressure, and heart disease. What was meant to aid survival

---

* There are two major types of cholesterol of clinical importance in our blood: LDL cholesterol and HDL cholesterol. Studies suggest that LDL cholesterol is bad, as it is associated with plaques in our arteries that increase our risk for heart disease. In contrast, HDL cholesterol is considered good, because it may reduce our risk for heart disease. People with metabolic syndrome typically have low concentrations of the good HDL cholesterol, while their levels of bad LDL cholesterol may or may not be elevated.

is now causing disease. Metabolic syndrome represents both nature's success and its failure.

This duality is good news, however. Because if we can understand what triggers the survival response in nature, we might obtain the clues we need to solve the riddle of obesity.

Metabolic syndrome represents both nature's success and its failure.

FOR ANIMALS IN NATURE, MAKING FAT IS PLANNED

Let's start by discussing how animals regulate their weight. You might think that fat carries such an advantage that an animal's natural instinct would be to eat whatever food is available to build up their fat stores. Yet this is not true.

Animals in the wild tend to stay at a specific weight. They will carry *some* extra fat for the unexpected emergency, but they will not become obese. If they eat a lot of food one day, they are likely to eat less the next, and as a result their weight remains within a desirable range. Laboratory studies show that if animals are forced to fast so that they lose weight, when the fasting stops they will eat enough to regain what they have lost. Likewise, if they are force-fed to make them gain weight, they tend to eat less until they have returned to their original weight when the force-feeding ends. One of the more interesting findings is that, in both situations, animals tend to return not to the weight they were after the altered feeding, but rather to what their weight would normally be at that time of the year. Their bodies seem to know what weight they're supposed to be.

While animals normally regulate their weight tightly, things change when an animal senses that food or water may soon become less available, such as when winter is approaching, or if they have to nest for a long period, or migrate a long distance. A month or two before the anticipated food shortage, the animal's behavior changes. It increases its foraging for food, and eats much more of it than usual, sometimes more than double. Its physiology changes, too, as we've discussed. It reduces how much energy it expends, becomes insulin resistant, and starts gaining fat, not just in its adipose tissue, but also in its blood and liver. It develops metabolic syndrome.

When it hibernates, a complete reversal occurs. The animal stops eating and lives off its fat, depending on it to provide the energy and water it needs. It initially stays insulin resistant so that the brain receives sufficient glucose. And when glucose stores eventually run low, leading blood levels to fall, it uses breakdown products from fat called **ketones** to fuel the brain.

During the fat-burning phase, animals appear calm and act as if they are not hungry. When the jungle fowl (a sort of wild chicken) is nesting, it won't eat even if food is brought over to it such that it does not have to leave its nest. Hibernating mammals that are awakened and offered food may take a bite or two, but generally show little interest. Hibernating squirrels that are woken up will not drink water. It is as if these animals have some sort of internal switch: when the switch is in one position, they eat excessive amounts of food and gain fat; when it is in the other, they lose their hunger and burn their fat.

This period of calm lasts only as long as they have fat to burn, however. Once fat supplies become low, the animal starts breaking down the protein in its muscle for energy. This triggers an alarm. The animal will wake from its sleep, or abandon its egg, to attempt to refuel; a migrating bird may collapse and fall into the sea.

This process—whereby animals maintain a weight within a narrow range until a challenge to their survival activates various biological processes that let them put on additional fat—I call the **survival switch**. While the process is turned on and off like a switch, it can also be adjusted high or low, like a dimmer switch. This switch is not unique to animals. Just as we humans share with animals the signs of metabolic syndrome, we also share that syndrome's cause. The same biological processes occur in us, where they have the same outcome: putting on fat.

THE SURVIVAL SWITCH: WHY HUMANS BECOME FAT

Historically, humans, like animals in the wild, have tended to maintain their weight. For many of us, it was easy to keep our weight within a narrow range early in life, regardless of what we ate. However, as I have gotten older, I know it has become easy for me to gain weight, but relatively hard to lose it. It is as if my body would prefer to be overweight. I do not think I am alone. All around the world, the majority of adults today are overweight or obese.

Why we are gaining weight? The *classical* teaching, which dates back to the 1920s, is that we are becoming overweight and developing diabetes because foods are now less expensive and readily available, and advances in transportation and other technologies have resulted in us exercising less and sitting more. The introduction of fast food, processed foods, and junk foods has made it easier to overeat, while elevators, escalators, trains, and automobiles have replaced the need to walk or bicycle. The internet, television, and smartphones have also made it easier and more enjoyable to stay home. The equation is simple physics: we are eating too much and exercising too little. When too much energy is produced (from food), and too little energy used (via exercise and other metabolic activities), the energy that is left over is stored as fat.

Consistent with the so-called "overnutrition" hypothesis is evidence that food portions have increased. Over the last century, the size of most soft drinks increased from 7 ounces to 10, 12, and even more. Restaurants keep increasing the size of meals, and all-you-can-eat buffets are common. Studies also show that the average number of daily calories people are eating has increased over the last decades. One analysis by the Food and Agricultural Organization of the United Nations reported that there was a more than 24 percent increase in total caloric intake between 1961 and 2013 (from about 2,900 calories a day to 3,600). People are also less active. Obesity correlates with the amount of time people spend watching television or are on the internet. Today the average person spends about ten or eleven hours on their cell phone or computer each day, but only about seventeen minutes exercising. No wonder we are getting fat.

There is a major problem with the overnutrition hypothesis, however. That problem is not its conclusion—that we are gaining weight because we are eating more while expending less energy—but rather that it blames this phenomenon solely on bad habits. Our culture does encourage us to eat more and not be active, and it is a contributing reason for the epidemic. However, as we learned from the survival switch, the root of the problem is *biological*.

The main reason people are eating more today is that many of us, and especially those of us who are overweight or obese, tend to be hungrier than usual because we do not get a sensation of being full after we have eaten. Normally, we get a sensation of **satiety** after a meal because a hormone called **leptin** tells a region in the brain called the hypothalamus to signal us to stop eating. Leptin is secreted by fat cells, and levels vary in relation to insulin levels and BMI. However, people who are overweight respond poorly to the leptin signal, something called **leptin resistance**, and so remain hungry longer. (This also explains why restaurants give us larger plates of food now than they did a few decades ago—not because they want us to feel we are getting a better deal, but because they know we will leave hungry if they don't.)

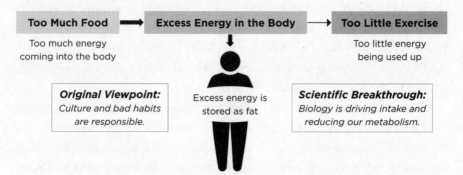

People are eating more and exercising less, and this is causing obesity—but not solely because of bad habits. Most people with obesity are resistant to leptin, impairing their ability to control their hunger, and many have reduced metabolism, especially at rest.

People who are overweight also do not burn fat as well as those without excess fat. (We will learn more about what causes this later.) Since they burn less fat, adipose tissue tends to accumulate. Meanwhile, when you burn less fat, you convert less stored energy to readily usable energy, or ATP. Your cells sense when ATP levels are low, and interpret this as a low-energy state despite the total energy in the cell, including that from fat, being normal or high. There is some evidence that this can cause fatigue, and also hunger. This compounds the effects of leptin resistance, causing you to eat even more food, until your ATP levels finally rise high enough that your hunger is satisfied. However, the cost is having eaten more food and made more fat.

This is the same biology that is observed in animals preparing for hibernation. In fact, the biology of animals that are putting on fat has remarkable similarities to that of the majority of humans who are struggling with their weight, suggesting that the underlying reason for human obesity is that we have turned

on the same survival switch used by animals in
nature. And if we can understand how we turned
on this switch, we would figure out the cause of
obesity—and, perhaps, how to cure it.

*It is not our culture
that is making us fat.
It is our biology.*

The evidence is overwhelming. The primary
reason we are becoming fat is not our culture.
It is our biology. Our culture is *responding to* our biology. Somehow, we have
unwittingly activated nature's survival switch. This is why we can lose weight
temporarily through dieting and exercise, but have trouble keeping it off.

With the survival switch activated, it is as if we are continuously preparing
for hibernation with no end in sight; unlike animals in the wild that turn this
switch off when they fast or hibernate, our switch appears permanently jammed
in the "on" position. And so long as this switch is on, we will continue to fight
a losing battle against obesity and its related diseases. The survival switch has
become a **fat switch**.

Yet, our detective work is paying off; it's given us significant insight already
into the biological process that is making us fat. Next, we need to figure out
what precisely triggers this switch and how it works.

CHAPTER 3

The Survival Switch

H ere's what we know so far: animals in the wild regulate their weight tightly, such that they only have a modest amount of fat. However, in preparation for situations in which food may not be available, many animals undergo a biological change in which they become excessively hungry and forage intently for food, while reducing energy expenditure when they rest. They maximize fat accumulation by increasing fat production and reducing the amount of fat burned, and they become insulin resistant to ensure sufficient glucose will be available for the brain. In essence, they initiate a comprehensive survival response that allows them to store enough fat to survive the winter in hibernation, or to migrate to a more hospitable environment.

A major question is what triggers this biologic response. The answer has evaded researchers throughout the world. Relatively little is known about what initiates the period of increased eating, and even less about what causes the animal to stop eating and start hibernating. Some researchers have suggested hibernation may be triggered by a fall in ambient temperature, or by changes in the length of day and night. Others have proposed that it may be triggered once an animal accumulates a certain level of fat. However, most studies suggest that the major stimulus for animals to begin hibernation is the unavailability of food or sometimes water, especially if temperatures have also dropped. Interestingly, there is also evidence that animals will further reduce

41

their metabolism shortly *before* they lower their body temperature and go into a deep sleep.

While there is much more to be learned about what turns the survival switch on and off for animals in the wild, I have an educated guess, based on the research, for what triggers it. Specifically, I believe that, at least in some animals, the survival program is initiated by eating a specific food with unique properties that extend beyond its caloric content. This special food is called fructose.

A BRIEF BUT NECESSARY FORAY INTO THE COMPLICATED TERMINOLOGY OF SUGARS

Fructose, the main sugar we'll be discussing here, is a type of carbohydrate. It is chemically similar to another commonly discussed sugar, **glucose**; both are "simple sugars," as they exist as single molecules. Fructose is commonly referred to as fruit sugar because it is the major sugar in fruit and honey and is the reason these foods taste sweet. Glucose, although it is also found in grains, beans, and vegetables, is sometimes referred to as blood sugar, as it is the major sugar found in our blood. It is also the main fuel used by the body.

Table sugar, or **sucrose**, is a "double sugar," formed from a fructose and a glucose molecule bonded together. This means that, when you eat table sugar, the bonds that hold fructose and glucose together must first be separated by an enzyme in the small intestine, allowing both single molecules to be absorbed separately. Fructose and glucose can also be mixed together, unbonded, to form a liquid known as **high-fructose corn syrup** (HFCS). The ratio of fructose to glucose in HFCS can vary, but HFCS tends to have a different ratio than table sugar, particularly in beverages, where it ranges from a 55:45 fructose:glucose ratio to as high as 65:35 in some fountain drinks. Most of the fructose that we eat comes not from fruit and honey but from table sugar or from HFCS added to foods; they are the two most common sources of added sugars.

There are also some sugars that do not contain fructose: for example, lactose (a combination of glucose and another simple sugar, galactose), the sugar present in milk. Also of note are **complex carbohydrates**, which are formed from chains of multiple sugar molecules bound together. While some complex carbohydrates are indigestible (we refer to these as fiber), others are digestible and make up a significant part of our diet. In plants these carbohydrates form various **starches**, while their counterpart in animals is called **glycogen**. Both starch and glycogen are made from chains of glucose, and neither contains fructose.

The word "sugar" can be confusing, as it is often used to refer to table sugar or sucrose, but it can also refer to sugars as a group. In this book, I will therefore try to be specific with the type of sugar I am discussing, especially when it comes to experimental studies. When we discuss the role of sugar in history and epidemiology, however, I may use sugar as another name for sucrose, and I will use the term **added sugars** when both sucrose and HFCS are being considered together.

FRUCTOSE TRIGGERS WEIGHT GAIN FOR ANIMALS IN THE WILD

Sometimes a single example can provide insights that help solve a problem, and for me the story of the hummingbird is that kind of example, as it provides important clues for what triggers the survival switch. The hummingbird has one of the fastest metabolisms of any animal alive. It breathes at an incredible rate of 250 times a minute, and its heart beats 1,200 times a minute. Its metabolism is so fast that its normal body temperature would be a fever for us: 102° Fahrenheit. With such a high metabolism, it seems impossible that this bird could become fat. That is, unless there were a mechanism that was simply so powerful that it could overwhelm even the most metabolically fit animal in the world.

Every morning, the hummingbird sets out on a mission to find flowers bearing the sweet nectar the bird craves. While hummingbirds may eat an occasional insect, nectar comprises the vast majority of their diet, and their appetite for it is voracious; it drinks as much as four times its weight in nectar per day. This leads to a remarkable increase in body fat, such that by early evening 40 percent of its overall weight may be fat. Its liver becomes so fatty that it is glistening and pearly white. The hummingbird does not simply become fat; it becomes diabetic. The glucose concentration in its blood can soar to levels of 700 milligrams per deciliter (mg/dL) or more, levels that would send us to the emergency room. By the end of the day, this bird we think of as lightweight and full of energy is fat and diabetic.

Yet the hummingbird never gets diabetes complications. Why? Because it burns off the fat and blood glucose overnight; by morning, both the fat and the diabetes have disappeared. The hummingbird's metabolism is so high that it needs this fat to survive while it sleeps. And if it runs out of fat stores during the night, it responds by slowing down its heart rate and breathing, much like a hibernating animal does. This allows the hummingbird to endure until the sun comes out and it can feed once more.

> By the end of every day, the hummingbird—a bird we think of as lightweight and full of energy—is fat and diabetic.

There must be something special about nectar that it can make a bird with super metabolism fat and diabetic in a single day. Nectar consists almost entirely of sugar water, and contains sucrose (which, as mentioned, is broken down into glucose and fructose in the gut), as well as "free" (unbonded) glucose and fructose—suggesting that it is one, or all, of these sugars that trigger weight gain and the other features of the survival switch.

Nectar is one of the few foods in nature that has a high sucrose content. The main sugar responsible for the sweetness of foods in the wild is fructose, the dominant sugar present in fruits and honey. And there is some evidence that animals prefer fructose-containing fruits and honey as a means for becoming fat.

One of the best examples are bears. During the fall, the American black bear and the grizzly bear both dramatically increase their food intake, often approaching 20,000 calories a day, which results in a daily weight gain of eight to ten pounds or more. One of their favorite foods is fruit. However, bears often do not eat fruit until late fall when it ripens, increasing the fruit's sugar content. Some studies show that the sugar content of fruit increases further following a morning frost, as occurs more frequently the closer it is to winter. A bear can eat an enormous amount of fruit in a very short time. One study found over sixty thousand Oregon grape seeds in one sample of bear scat, which is consistent with the bear having eaten approximately ten thousand grapes during the prior twenty-four to forty-eight hours. Black bears and grizzly bears—as well as other bears, including the sloth bear of Indonesia and the sun bear of Borneo—also seek honey. You may recall the children's character Winnie the Pooh, a fat and cuddly teddy bear that lived in the Hundred Acre Wood and loved honey. Bears do love honey, and use it as a food source to gain weight before they hibernate.

Other animals also eat fruit as a means to gain fat prior to hibernation. In Madagascar there is a fat-tailed dwarf lemur that hibernates in warm weather (something technically called **estivation**, meaning "to pass the summer"). During Madagascar's dry season, there can be severe droughts. To prepare for this, the lemur will eat huge amounts of fruit during the wet season, gaining fat that it stores in its tail. Then, when the dry season comes, it will hole up in a tree hollow, drop its body temperature, and go into a deep sleep for up to six months, living off the calories and water produced as it slowly burns the fat off.

Many migrating birds switch from an insect-based diet to a fruit-based diet in autumn before they fly south for the winter. Experimental studies have shown that this switch is associated with a dramatic increase in total caloric intake, a 30 percent fall in metabolic rate when at rest, and remarkable weight gains, primarily from fat. We have previously mentioned the pacu fish, which, along with other fruit-eating fish, lives off ripe fruit that drops into the Amazon during yearly floods.

All of this suggests that something present in fruit may be a means for triggering weight gain and fat accumulation. Paired with what we know about hummingbirds, fructose seems the most likely culprit. But is there more direct evidence?

EARLY RESEARCH INTO FRUCTOSE

Observations in nature are important, but there are many variables that one cannot control for. While fructose is fruit's main nutrient, it also contains multiple other substances that could have biological effects. To find out if fructose really is triggering the survival switch, it is important to look at, and do, experiments in a controlled laboratory setting.

Studies as early as the 1950s showed that fructose was much more effective, compared to glucose, in causing prediabetes (we now call this insulin resistance) in laboratory animals. Further studies in the 1970s and 1980s provided more ammunition, demonstrating that fructose also seemed to have the ability to increase triglycerides in the blood and to stimulate weight gain. However, very few studies of fructose were performed aside from these, and by the turn of the twenty-first century, fructose as a potential cause of obesity had fallen off the radar.

Indeed, there was little interest in sucrose or fructose in the medical world until the late 1990s. The prevailing belief was that these sugars were "empty calories," meaning that they had very little nutritional value but were otherwise safe. Sugars are carbohydrates, which contain only 4 calories per gram, and so were not considered to be as likely to cause weight gain as fat, which has more than twice the number of calories, with 9 per gram.*

Nevertheless, a small group of researchers remained concerned that sugar might be more important as a cause of obesity than commonly thought. Research into this viewpoint was further stimulated by a provocative 2004 paper by several leading authors in the obesity field that noted a further rise in the frequency of obesity following the introduction of HFCS. Around the same time, a low-carbohydrate diet introduced by Robert Atkins was becoming increasingly popular as a means to lose weight. Since all sugars are carbohydrates, the Atkins diet also restricted the intake of HFCS and fructose generally.

The interest in HFCS as a potential cause of obesity rekindled interest in fructose, and soon there were reports that not only did fructose cause insulin

---

* Calories are units of energy defined as the amount of heat required to warm water by 1 degree Celsius. It is the common way to measure the amount of energy in food. When we use the word "calories," it is actually kilocalories, one thousand of these units of heat. However, calorie is the commonly used term.

resistance and an elevation in blood triglycerides in laboratory animals, but it also could cause other features of metabolic syndrome, including obesity (particularly increased abdominal fat), elevated blood pressure, and fatty liver.

It was around that time, in 2004, that my research group, then at the University of Florida, began studying fructose. We actually entered this topic by accident, as our primary interest was in a substance known as **uric acid**. Widely considered a waste product, uric acid is generated during normal metabolism, and our body eliminates it largely by excreting it in our urine, though some is also disposed of in the gut, where bacteria breaks it down. However, levels of uric acid can build up in the blood; we see this especially in people who are overweight and/or have prediabetes. When levels get too high, the uric acid becomes unstable and can crystallize, especially in the joints. This results in local inflammation that causes a painful arthritis known as **gout**.

Our group discovered that uric acid was not simply a waste product; it was biologically active. One of our findings was that raising uric acid levels could increase blood pressure. This made me wonder if uric acid might have a role in hypertension, and in turn, what caused high uric acid levels, especially given the evidence that our uric acid levels had been increasing in parallel with the rise in hypertension and obesity throughout the twentieth century. A logical possibility was that it related to diet; it was well known that both alcohol and red meats can raise uric acid levels. However, red meat intake had not increased much during this time, raising the possibility that another food might be to blame.

One possibility was sugar. Doctors had known since the 1800s that both table sugar and fruit could also cause gout attacks, and by the 1970s, studies had been done demonstrating that fructose was unique among sugars in its ability to raise uric acid. This led me to wonder if fructose intake might increase blood pressure through its ability to raise uric acid levels.

To study this, Takahiko Nakagawa from our research group gave fructose plus **allopurinol**, a drug that blocks uric acid production, to half of a group of laboratory rats; the other half received only fructose. The animals that received only fructose gained weight; developed insulin resistance, elevated blood triglycerides, and high uric acid levels; and became hypertensive. The rats that also received allopurinol did not experience an increase in uric acid or develop high blood pressure, as we predicted. But there was an additional, unexpected twist: the allopurinol blocked not only the development of hypertension, but also, partially, the weight gain, insulin resistance, and rise in blood triglycerides.

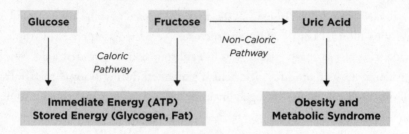

A mystery: How could uric acid have a role in obesity when it is not involved in the generation of energy from fructose?

The observation that uric acid had a role in how fructose caused obesity was surprising, for uric acid was thought to be an unrelated side effect of fructose metabolism. Indeed, the general belief was that fructose was metabolized like glucose: that once it was broken down, its by-products were used to generate energy that was either used immediately or stored as fat (or glycogen; as mentioned, a form of short-term storage for carbohydrates). In other words, many scientists thought that fructose increased fat because of its caloric content—but this theory could not explain why blocking the production of uric acid would protect an animal from obesity and insulin resistance.

I realized that fructose's role in metabolic syndrome was not fully understood. As Sherlock might have said, there was a mystery afoot. For the last twenty years, our research group, as well as others, has attempted to crack the problem of how fructose activates the survival switch and the role of uric acid in this process. To better explain our work, I will take us through many of the questions we asked and the experiments we performed to investigate this mystery.

DOES FRUCTOSE CAUSE METABOLIC SYNDROME?

Early on, we wanted to determine in our own laboratory whether fructose intake could truly mimic what animals do when they prepare for hibernation.

We found that there was some variability in how mice and rats responded to fructose in our experiments, but that the most effective way to induce obesity was to provide fructose in drinking water, as opposed to putting it in food. Giving fructose in water also provided another advantage: we could separate food intake from fructose intake. In other words, we could see how drinking fructose affected intake of foods that did not themselves contain fructose.

Normally, if you give an animal a high-calorie drink, they will reduce the amount of food they eat so that their overall calorie intake stays the same. When laboratory mice were given fructose in their drinking water, they initially compensated for the calories they were getting from fructose by decreasing their food intake. However, after several weeks, this pattern changed. They not only continued to drink the same amount of fructose, or even more, but also *increased* their food intake, so that their overall caloric intake was significantly higher than that of the control group drinking regular water. In essence, they acted persistently hungry. They also became less active (which we measured using laser lights that detect movement), and literally started to lie around. After several months, they had gained a lot more fat compared to the control mice, on their abdomens in particular, and had developed fatty liver and insulin resistance. In contrast, the control mice remained healthy and lean. Specific analyses further showed that the fructose-drinking mice not only ate more calories overall, but also had decreased their metabolism when they were at rest. They started accumulating fat not only due to increased production of fat, but also because they were burning less fat.

In other studies performed in laboratory rats, we confirmed that intake of a high-fructose diet caused weight gain, fat accumulation, fatty liver, and insulin resistance. Our group and other researchers found that high fructose intake leads to elevated blood pressure, high blood triglycerides, and markers of inflammation. Additionally, several other groups found that high fructose intake reduced HDL cholesterol (the good cholesterol). In short, fructose intake could cause every single feature of metabolic syndrome.

Nutrition scientists Kimber Stanhope and Peter Havel at the University of California, Davis observed similar findings in a study of overweight volunteers in which subjects randomly received beverages containing either fructose or glucose for ten weeks. Both groups ate more food than expected for their calculated energy needs, resulting in a similar increase in weight: three pounds.

Animals may dramatically increase their intake of fruits and honey in the fall not because these foods are an available source of calories, but because they are important to triggering the survival switch.

However, the group given fructose beverages developed much worse features of metabolic syndrome than the group given glucose, including more abdominal fat, more insulin resistance, lower energy metabolism at rest, higher blood levels of triglycerides and uric acid, and even signs that fatty liver was developing, as indicated by abnormal liver function tests. Many of these features, such as elevated triglycerides, elevated uric acid, and lower energy metabolism, were more pronounced after meals.

The data is clear: excessive intake of fructose stimulates food intake and the development of metabolic syndrome in both animals and humans. Animals may dramatically increase their intake of fruits and honey in the fall not because these foods are an available source of calories; rather, the fructose present in these foods may be important to disengaging the normal regulation of weight and triggering the survival switch.

HOW DOES FRUCTOSE CAUSE METABOLIC SYNDROME? IS IT DEPENDENT ON CALORIES?

As mentioned, the animals in our studies initially compensated for greater fructose intake by eating less food, but after several weeks, the animals began eating more and more food, as though continually hungry. In addition, their resting metabolism fell. This is similar to the changes observed in society as a whole over the past few decades: we are eating more while expending less energy. Could this be how fructose causes metabolic syndrome? By making us hungry, which leads us to eat more than we should, while reducing our metabolism?

One way to test this is to see if fructose causes metabolic syndrome when calories are restricted. In other words, do not let fructose-fed animals eat additional food, even when their hunger tells them they should. We designed multiple studies that provided the same total number of calories to two groups of rats, one given fructose and one not. The findings were always the same: fructose causes weight gain primarily by stimulating calorie intake. That is, in the absence of increased food intake, weight gain is minimal.*

While we found no difference between the two groups in weight gain in animals fed the same number of calories, other differences were impressive. Features of metabolic syndrome such as insulin resistance, elevated blood triglycerides, and elevated blood pressure still developed in the fructose-fed rats, but were absent in the control rats.

While we have shown this multiple times using fructose as the dietary sugar, a great example comes from a study performed in my laboratory by Carlos Roncal using sucrose (table sugar; as noted, a combination of fructose and glucose). Carlos placed one group of rats on a diet containing 40 percent sucrose, and a second group on the same diet, but with the sucrose replaced by starch (a complex carbohydrate that contains no fructose). To ensure all animals ate the same amount, every day he would measure how much food the animals had consumed, then base the decision of how much food to give the next day on the animal that had eaten the least.

As Carlos and I were running the experiment, we did not notice that one rat tended to eat very little, so the experiment continued for four months with all the animals eating the same amount of food as the rat with the poor appetite. It eventually became apparent to us that this one rat had cancer, and consequently, all our animals had been on a particularly stringent diet. This unplanned event turned out to be fortunate, for we had unwittingly performed an ideal study to determine if sucrose had metabolic effects even when food intake was low.

At the end of the experiment, we had a striking finding. Despite the calorie restriction, the sucrose-fed rats had all developed diabetes, and their livers were filled with fat. In contrast, the starch-fed rats had normal-appearing livers, and none had diabetes. As far as weight was concerned, the animals that had received sucrose tended to weigh more than the starch-fed rats, but not significantly so. This latter finding made sense, as it was consistent with our other

---

* Although stimulation of food intake is the main reason fructose causes weight gain, we did see some weight gain in our studies due to lower metabolism. This gain was not significant, but this may have been because most of our studies were short-term and limited to weeks or only a few months. It is quite possible that weight differences would have been larger were the diets maintained over many months.

Fructose causes weight gain by encouraging increased food intake, but causes the other features of metabolic syndrome even when food intake remains the same.

studies showing that much of the weight gain in a high-sugar diet is driven by calories (although a little is due to the decrease in energy being burned).

The HFCS industry claims we are getting fat because we are eating too much and exercising too little, and that it has nothing to do with *what* we are eating—specifically, with our high intake of added sugars. They have sponsored research that has concluded there is no difference in weight gain between individuals receiving a diet high in fructose and a control diet, so long as caloric intake is equal. This makes you think that HFCS and sucrose are not the culprits driving the obesity epidemic. However, they fail to consider that *the way* sucrose and HFCS cause weight gain is by activating a biological process that makes you persistently hungry and drives you to eat more. Further, they did not investigate other characteristics of metabolic syndrome (abdominal fat accumulation, insulin resistance, fatty liver, etc.) that are driven by fructose independently of caloric intake.

This leads us to a new question: What is it about fructose that makes us want to eat more?

HOW DOES FRUCTOSE DRIVE HUNGER?

One of the main ways animals control their weight is through the actions of a hormone known as leptin. Leptin, which you'll recall is released from fat cells, is what tells our brain we are full. However, it has been shown that, when gaining weight in preparation for hibernation in the fall, bears become resistant to leptin's effects. People who are overweight or obese also are commonly resistant to leptin. This leptin resistance results in persistent hunger, such that bears and people alike eat more than they need, resulting in weight gain.

Our research group, working with physiologist Philip Scarpace, was able to show that when animals in the lab are given a high-fructose diet, they become leptin resistant, although it can take several weeks to months. Once the animals are leptin resistant, they get hungrier, eat more food than they need, and gain weight. Notably, the leptin resistance also persists for several weeks *after* the fructose in their diet is taken away.

There are two caveats here worth highlighting. First, being leptin resistant by itself does not mean you will gain weight. If you are leptin resistant but do not consume additional calories, either because food is not available or because you are able to overcome the biological impulse to eat (a difficult thing to do!), you will not gain weight; you will simply stay hungry. Second, the amount of weight you gain when you are leptin resistant depends on the type of food you eat. For example, if the food you eat is high in calories, as with fatty foods, you will gain more than if the food is low in calories.

The phenomenon of leptin resistance explains why feeding a high-fat diet to animals on fructose can cause dramatic weight gain. It also explains why a high-fat diet in the absence of fructose does not cause weight gain: the animals remain sensitive to the effects of leptin, and regulate their food intake accordingly.* This is the likely explanation for why popular high-fat, low-carb diets do not cause obesity.

> *Fructose causes leptin resistance, which makes us hungrier, which leads us to eat more and gain weight.*

Fructose causes leptin resistance, which makes us hungrier, which leads us to eat more. But is that the only role fructose plays in weight gain? Most of us love sweet foods; many people claim to crave them. Does this love and craving for sweets have any influence on our food intake?

---

* We previously showed that a diet high in lard does not cause weight gain in laboratory animals if no fructose is present. However, a diet enriched in butter does appear to cause some weight gain, although without activating the survival switch. The mechanism is unclear, but might relate to other contents in butter or to the enclosure effect (see chapter nine).

DOES OUR LOVE AND CRAVING FOR SWEETS PLAY A ROLE IN HOW FRUCTOSE CAUSES OBESITY?

You could say we have a bit of a love affair with sugar, for when we eat sweet foods, it triggers the release of **dopamine** in our brain that provides a sense of pleasure. There is even some evidence that our liking for sugar can progress to a craving that can resemble addiction (a topic we'll discuss further in chapter seven). For example, mice that are provided water with sucrose intermittently drink it very fast whenever it is available, and show signs of anxiety and withdrawal when the sugar water is withheld. This raises the question of whether our love of sugar might also have a role in causing obesity, in addition to the development of leptin resistance.

To investigate, our research group performed a study with fellow University of Colorado researchers Tom Finger and Sue Kinnamon to evaluate whether fructose would cause obesity in mice that had been genetically engineered to lack all sense of taste (so-called **knockout** mice, as the genes for taste have been "knocked out" of their DNA). Interestingly, these "taste-blind" mice still preferred drinks that contained fructose, as well as drinks that contained sucrose and HFCS, compared to water alone. They also still developed all of the features of metabolic syndrome. Not surprisingly, this was also associated with the development of leptin resistance.

Our taste for sugar encourages us to eat more of it, but we would get fat from sugar even if we could not taste it.

We also looked at whether there was a difference between taste-blind mice and normal mice when it came to how much fructose they chose to consume. While both taste-blind mice and normal mice preferred fructose over water, the normal mice did drink *more* fructose, suggesting that the main effect of sweet taste is to encourage intake of sweet foods.* Both groups of mice also got fat—although, quite unexpectedly, the

---

* If you're wondering about artificial sweeteners, they also stimulate the sweet taste receptors in the tongue, and, as one would predict, encourage intake of sweets. Unlike fructose, however, they alone do not cause obesity. See chapter eight for more.

normal mice gained less weight than the taste-blind mice—even though the normal mice ate more fructose. (This turned out to be because the taste-blind mice developed more severe leptin resistance, although the reason they did so remains unknown.) This suggests that, while our taste for sugar does encourage us to eat more of it, we would get fat from sugar even if we could not taste it.

While we think of the sweet taste as a major reason why we like sugar and HFCS (as well as fructose), the observation that taste-blind mice still prefer fructose over water suggests that our liking for fructose might involve other mechanisms besides taste. This conclusion was further supported by a study from another research team, who were studying mice that had been modified so that they could not taste sweetness but still had their other tastes intact. These mice continued to like sucrose and still experienced a dopamine response in their brains when consuming it. But while artificial sugars, such as sucralose, also generated a dopamine response in normal mice, the mice that could not taste sweetness no longer had a dopamine response. They also did not demonstrate any preference for it over regular water, the way the normal mice did. So there is something special about sucrose that results in pleasure even when its sweetness cannot be tasted.

One possibility for why our craving for fructose-containing sugars persists even when we cannot taste them is that the craving is related instead to how fructose is metabolized (that is, how it is broken down in the body). As mentioned earlier in this chapter, fructose and glucose are metabolized in much the same way, but there are some differences. Fructose is broken down into uric acid, for example.

Our research group therefore wanted to determine whether there was something special about how fructose was metabolized that could explain why we crave fructose-containing sugars, and whether this had anything to do with how fructose causes metabolic syndrome.

Fructose is initially broken down by a special enzyme called **fructokinase**. We were able to obtain mice that had been genetically modified not to produce fructokinase. These mice could still taste the sweetness of sugar and metabolize fructose using the same enzyme used for glucose. But the special system designed to only metabolize fructose, the primary one through which most fructose is broken down, was fully blocked.

We next offered these special mice a choice of drinking regular water or water containing different types of sugar. Our findings were very exciting. These special mice did not prefer fructose water over regular water, even though they did prefer glucose water. Moreover, they were completely protected from obesity and metabolic syndrome, even if they were forced to drink large amounts of fructose. They also fully controlled their food intake and stayed lean to a very old age (which we later showed was because they remained sensitive to leptin).

One of the special things about fructokinase is where it is found in the body: it is primarily concentrated in the liver, intestines, and kidneys, and, to a lesser extent, the brain. This made us wonder if fructose's ability to cause obesity and metabolic syndrome was driven by the metabolism of fructose in one of these organs.

To study this, Miguel Lanaspa from our research group performed a set of experiments that gave new insights into both the source of our fructose craving and how fructose drives obesity and metabolic syndrome. By blocking fructose metabolism in specific organs in mice, while allowing fructose to be metabolized in other organs, he discovered that it was the liver that was fully responsible for how fructose causes obesity and metabolic syndrome. This is not so surprising, in retrospect, since the liver is the main organ that metabolizes the foods we eat. When he blocked fructose metabolism in the liver, the mice stayed lean and maintained normal leptin signaling to the brain.

The metabolism of fructose controls our preference for sugar as well as how fructose causes obesity and metabolic syndrome.

Interestingly, the mice that couldn't metabolize fructose in the liver continued to love fructose, sucrose, and HFCS and to drink excessive amounts of water containing these sugars. In contrast, mice unable to metabolize fructose in the gut drank minimal water with fructose-containing sugars, suggesting that the preference for fructose may relate to some type of intestine–brain communication. And notably, when these latter mice were forced to eat fructose anyway, they developed obesity and metabolic syndrome.

What these studies suggest is that the metabolism of fructose through this special enzyme, fructokinase, may explain both why we prefer sugar *and* how fructose causes obesity and metabolic syndrome, but also that it does these two things through separate areas of the body. The preference for sugar is dependent on metabolism of fructose in the intestines, while fructose's ability to cause obesity and insulin resistance stems from its metabolism in the liver.

THE MILLION-DOLLAR QUESTION: HOW DOES FRUCTOSE ACTIVATE THE SURVIVAL SWITCH?

The question we were left with, then, was: What is it about the metabolism of fructose that activates the survival switch? The answer turns out to be related to energy.

Recall that when we eat, the calories in our food are either turned into usable energy or stored for later use. The usable form of energy is called **ATP**, short for **adenosine triphosphate**. Most of our ATP is made in energy factories known as mitochondria. Energy can also be stored as fat or glycogen (the storage form of carbohydrates), both of which can be converted to ATP if food is not available. Whether it is getting its ATP from food metabolism or from stored fat or glycogen, the body has to maintain a certain level in order to respond rapidly to its energy needs, such as running, thinking, or even sleeping.

ATP is also required to metabolize food. This energy expenditure is worthwhile, because food generates much more ATP than is used up to metabolize it. However, because the metabolism does use *some* ATP, levels of ATP in our cells (and especially the liver) could theoretically fall below the body's preferred level prior to the completion of metabolism and its generation of more ATP. Fortunately, for the metabolism of most foods, there is a check-and-balance system that prevents this from happening. Take glucose. If ATP levels start to fall while glucose is being metabolized, the whole system slows down or stops until the ATP is replenished. As a result, ATP levels never fall significantly and all remains well.

Fructose metabolism is different. There is no check-and-balance system that protects the liver or other organs if ATP levels fall. Fructokinase breaks down fructose very rapidly, quickly using up ATP in the process, and so ATP levels can fall precipitously if a lot of fructose is being metabolized.

The initial fall in ATP that occurs during fructose metabolism causes a chain reaction that keeps energy levels low. When ATP is used for energy, it gives up a phosphate to become ADP (adenosine diphosphate). ADP can be converted back to ATP, and this is what normally happens during the metabolism of glucose and other nutrients. However, when fructose is metabolized, the ADP is broken down into **AMP (adenosine monophosphate)**, and then further metabolized to make uric acid. As ADP and AMP are removed to generate uric acid, the cell's ability to remake ATP becomes impaired.

This is not the only way that fructose metabolism affects energy levels, however. You may recall from the beginning of this chapter that my interest in fructose began when we discovered that lowering uric acid could partially block fructose's ability to cause metabolic syndrome. At the time, it was unclear how this worked.

We subsequently learned that the uric acid formed from AMP also affects ATP levels in its own right. Specifically, it causes oxidative stress to the mitochondria, which further reduces their ability to make ATP while stimulating the production of fat. The oxidative stress caused by uric acid also blocks the burning of fatty acids released from stored fat. The net effect is that not only do the mitochondria make less ATP, but also the calories that would have been used to make ATP are now being stored as body fat.

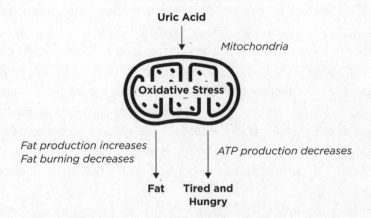

Uric acid causes oxidative stress to the mitochondria, decreasing energy production, impairing fat burning, and stimulating fat production.

When ATP levels fall in the cell, the body treats it as an emergency. It responds by stimulating hunger immediately.* This leads to increased food intake aimed at restoring ATP levels, among other biologic effects. However, due to the ongoing oxidative stress in the mitochondria, much of the calories end up being converted to fat—and if the food ingested includes fructose, it only exacerbates the issue, dropping ATP levels further and creating additional oxidative stress. Eventually, ATP levels recover, but by the time they do, much of the food we have eaten has been converted to fat.

A FULLER CHARACTERIZATION OF THE SURVIVAL SWITCH TRIGGERED BY FRUCTOSE

In short, the way fructose works is that it mimics starvation by creating a low-energy state inside our cells, signaling to the body that there is an energy crisis. This is what flips the survival switch to the "on" position.

The more we have studied this biological response to fructose, the more apparent it has become that its purpose is to aid survival. Listed below are the major effects of fructose that have been discovered, most of which stem from the decrease in energy and generation of uric acid that occurs when fructose is metabolized. Many of these will be discussed in more detail later.

The Survival Switch	
Hunger	Driven by low ATP levels, which simulates starvation, and by leptin resistance, which prevents us from recognizing when we are full.
Craving	Driven by fructose metabolism in the intestines and possibly the brain.
Foraging behavior	Aids in the search for food in unfamiliar areas. Includes risk taking, impulsiveness, rapid decision making, and aggression.

---

* Notably, while these acute changes in ATP do have a role in stimulating food intake, leptin resistance, which develops over time, remains the more important mechanism for stimulating food intake and weight gain.

Increased food intake	Driven by hunger and craving, and achieved through foraging behavior.
Reduced metabolism when at rest	Allows the body to conserve energy when not needed for foraging. Likely from effects on mitochondrial function.
Fat accumulation	The result of a combination of increased production and decreased burning of fat. Caused by oxidative stress to the mitochondria, especially in the liver. Provides a source of stored energy and metabolic water.
Glycogen accumulation	Produced in the liver alongside fat with activation of the survival switch. Provides another source of stored energy and metabolic water, similar to fat. Unlike fat, it contains water (in addition to making water when metabolized), which it obtains from the blood.
Thirst	Likely stimulated by increased glycogen production, which simulates dehydration when removing water from the blood.
Insulin resistance	Makes more glucose available to the brain to fuel the quick decisions required to survive while foraging. Linked with oxidative stress to the mitochondria.
Increased blood pressure	Maintains circulation in case of dehydration or low availability of salt. Driven in part by the effects of uric acid.
Salt retention	Supports circulation. Driven by the effects of fructose on the kidney.
Low-grade inflammation	Provides some defense against infection, such as malaria. Likely driven in part by the effects of uric acid.
Reduced oxygen needs	Helps animals survive when oxygen levels are low. The metabolism of fructose depresses mitochondrial function and shifts energy production to a more primitive system, glycolysis, that does not require oxygen the way it does in the mitochondria.

Mother Nature is smart. Consuming fructose tricks an animal into thinking its energy stores are low, even when it has plenty of untapped energy in the form of fat. This drives the animal to increase its fat stores and triggers a host of other metabolic responses that aid survival in a crisis. It is a brilliant system, as it allows an animal to put on fat *before* it is in trouble, rather than having to figure out how to survive once no food or water is available.

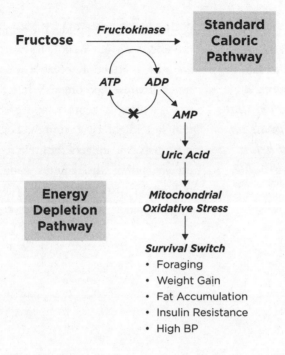

The main way fructose is metabolized is by an enzyme called fructokinase. This enzyme uses ATP, which generates ADP. While ADP is commonly remade into ATP, this regeneration of ATP is reduced because other chemical reactions stimulated during the metabolism of fructose drive the conversion of AMP to uric acid. In turn, the uric acid causes oxidative stress to the mitochondria that trigger the survival switch. This occurs independently of the stepwise breakdown of fructose that occurs with standard carbohydrate metabolism.

In nature, fructose is part of a broader interdependent system in which plants and animals help each other to survive. The flowers generate sugary nectar that encourages the hummingbird to visit, which in turn provides a vehicle for the plant to spread its pollen to other flowers for reproduction. The fruit of trees in the Amazon jungle ripens synchronous with the yearly floods, which not only supplies the pacu fish with food, but also aids the trees by dispersing their seeds through the fish's excrement. Likewise, the maturation of fruit in the late summer and fall provides ripe, fructose-rich fruit for migratory birds and hibernating animals, helping them increase their fat stores before winter hits while aiding the dispersal and planting of seeds ahead of the spring.

We have disrupted this beautiful balance by finding ways to eat fructose all year long. The dream system designed by Mother Nature appears to have failed

Fructose tricks the body into increasing its fat stores, a brilliant system that allows animals to put on fat before they get in trouble.

us. But before we consider the details of how, and the effects on our health, it's worth pausing to ask why. Is it simply because we are eating too much fructose, too often? While this is a major reason, there is another, as we shall see—one that just might be a surprise. For, unlike most mammals, we are very sensitive to fructose, and understanding why requires going back in time millions of years to investigate yet another mystery in biology.

CHAPTER 4

Why We Are Becoming Fat

Of all animals, humans and their primate cousins have one of the strongest love affairs with fructose, the main sugar present in fruit. For apes, fruit is not just their favorite food; it is something they crave. A study in Indonesia found that orangutans living in the tropical rain forests gorge on fruit during the few months when it is widely available, consuming it exclusively. During this time, they double their normal intake of calories and see a marked increase in body fat. For the rest of the year, they subsist mostly on bark and leaves, and end up surviving largely by burning the fat they accumulated when fruit was more available. Other apes also rely on ripe fruits for valuable calories. Chimpanzees, for example, especially love figs, which are often available throughout the year.

Our love affair with fructose has deep roots, for fructose saved our shared ancestors from extinction more than once. At least two times in our history, our survival was linked not simply with fructose, but with lifesaving genetic mutations that gave us a winning combination: the ability to store *more* fat from *less* fructose. These mutations, random events that just happened to provide a critical survival advantage that saved us from extinction, could be considered miracles. However, these miracles come with a twist, for ironically, these same mutations are now a big part of the reason we humans are getting fat.

AN ASTEROID, AN EXTINCTION, AND A MIRACLE

Millions and millions of years ago, astronomers believe, an asteroid collision in the belt between Mars and Jupiter ejected rock fragments, one of which found its way to Earth to cause one of the greatest extinctions of all time. Once the asteroid hit our atmosphere, it became a flaming meteorite, called Chixculub, after a Maya town close to where the impact site was discovered. It is thought this fireball hit the Yucatán around 65 million years ago, at the end of the Cretaceous Period, during which dinosaurs still ruled the planet. The meteorite was enormous, six to ten miles in diameter, and crashed into Earth at a speed of about 50,000 miles per hour, resulting in a crater sixty miles in diameter and eighteen miles deep. The impact caused a massive tsunami and earthquakes with magnitudes greater than 10, releasing more than a billion times the energy of an atomic bomb. Dust, dirt, and rock were thrown high into the air, to such a level that sunlight was blocked for a year or more. Initially there was massive heat and wildfire, but this was rapidly followed by prolonged night due to the atmospheric dust. This resulted in what's called an "impact winter," where temperatures fell a mean of 7° Celsius. With minimal sunlight, plants died and food became scarce.

It was a desperate time for life on Earth. Nearly 75 percent of all animal species became extinct, including the dinosaurs. The remaining species suffered terrible losses, with few surviving.

Among the survivors were some small mammals, including the earliest primates. Genetic studies suggest that these early primates had been around for about 5 million years before the impact and were of two types: the ancestors of lemurs, those small, cute, wet-nosed, big-eyed primates living in Madagascar; and the ancestors of dry-nosed primates like monkeys, apes, and humans. It is thought that these nimble animals lived primarily on fruit, and so their existence must have been precarious, for fruit was hard to find. How did these primates survive?

My interest in this mass extinction event began when I learned that the DNA of today's dry-nosed primates contains a mutation that knocked out our ability to make our own vitamin C. The exact timing of the mutation is not precisely known, but there is evidence that it occurred around the time of the impact. That this mutation took over the entire population of dry-nosed primates suggests it must have provided a survival advantage. But what was that advantage?

Vitamin C is an antioxidant, meaning it protects the body from oxidative stress, and is important for a lot of biological functions. If a person doesn't get enough vitamin C, they can get sick with scurvy. People with scurvy suffer from fatigue, bleeding gums, and joint pain, and it frequently affected sailors before a ship's physician by the name of James Lind discovered that it could be treated by eating fruit. (This led to the practice of giving limes and lemons to sailors when they were at sea, and is why "limey" became a nickname for British sailors.)

Given vitamin C's importance, why would a mutation that removed our ability to make it be beneficial? Especially in the aftermath of a meteorite impact, when the main dietary source of vitamin C was fruit, and fruit was almost certainly hard to find? It seems incongruous that losing the ability to combat oxidative stress would be a good thing during such a massive disaster. That is, of course, unless oxidative stress was, for some reason, desirable!

Recall that when we consume fructose, uric acid is generated, and that uric acid exerts oxidative stress on our energy factories, the mitochondria. This oxidative stress reduces the production of ATP and shunts the calories instead to fat. It also causes us to burn less fat, which further reduces metabolism. Hence, oxidative stress is important in how fructose increases body fat, which aids survival when food is not available. And too much vitamin C, which blocks oxidative stress, might be predicted to dampen this survival switch, leading to less production of fat.

Fruit contains vitamin C, but as fruit matures, its vitamin C content falls, while the fructose content increases. Fruit contains the most fructose and the least vitamin C when it is mature and its seeds are ready to be planted. This high fructose level is likely the reason animals tend to favor eating ripe fruit; it provides the best raw materials for driving fat storage.

However, if an animal also makes its own vitamin C, then the effect of even ripe fruit on stimulating fat production might be hindered, depending on how high the animal's vitamin C levels were. And if an animal were starving, low vitamin C levels would be ideal, in order to maximize fat production in response to fructose. Miguel Lanaspa and I therefore wondered if the inability to make vitamin C might have provided a survival advantage to our primate ancestors, by enhancing the ability of fructose to increase body fat at a time when animals struggled to find enough to eat.

To study the effect of vitamin C on fat, we used mice that had been genetically altered so that they were unable to make vitamin C, similar to humans today. Just like us, these modified animals require vitamin C in their diet, or else they can get very sick. By using these mice, we could control how much vitamin C each mouse received. We separated the mice into two groups, each of which received either a low or high dose of vitamin C, and then gave them drinking water that had been spiked with HFCS so its sugar content was similar to that of a soft drink. All of the mice loved the sweetened water, and both groups drank the same amount. However, the mice on the low dose of vitamin C became fatter than those receiving the high dose.

Today, the loss of our ability to make vitamin C has made us more susceptible to becoming fat from fructose.

The loss of the ability to make vitamin C was beneficial for early primates struggling to survive the great extinction that killed the dinosaurs because it allowed them to generate more fat despite dwindling amounts of fruit. Today, however, the loss of vitamin C makes us more susceptible to sugar's fat-storage effects. Indeed, many studies have confirmed that overweight people tend to have low vitamin C levels in their blood. There are also many intriguing pilot studies showing that administering vitamin C can improve features of metabolic syndrome in both animals and humans. (We will discuss the role of vitamin C in both preventing and treating obesity further in chapters nine and ten.)

The asteroid impact was not the only threat to the survival of our species. There was a second extinction event that we also narrowly escaped, and that, ironically, also increased our risk for obesity today.

HOW THE FIG AND THE FIG WASP
INFLUENCED OUR RISK FOR BECOMING FAT

Around 24 million years ago, the first ape appeared in East Africa. The ape represented a major evolutionary breakthrough compared to its monkey cousins, for it had a larger head and body, and also no tail. This early ape lived in the rain forest, where it stayed in the canopy and ate a diet primarily of fruits.

The climate in Africa during the early Miocene Epoch was a tropical paradise, with fruit available all year long and relatively few predators, and within just a few million years, the ape population had expanded into more than ten different species. Then, around 17 million years ago, global temperatures slowly began to decrease, likely from volcanic activity in the Rift Valley. Ice accumulated at the poles, and ocean levels started falling. The Sahara, which had been underwater, turned into a swamp, and Africa, previously separated from Eurasia by water, became connected by a land bridge.

The development of a land highway to Eurasia allowed many animals to enter what is now the Middle East and Asia Minor, including elephants, rhinos, giraffes, and even anteaters. Among the travelers were several species of apes, which found the woodlands and forests of their new environment quite hospitable. Soon there were colonies of apes living in what is now the Middle East and Europe.

The world continued to cool. In Europe, this was associated with seasonal monsoons followed by mild winters, and a change in habitat in which forests thinned and open grasslands formed. Fruit became less available, and as the climate continued to worsen over the next several million years, the European apes had to become more resourceful. This required coming out of the trees to look for alternative foods such as roots and tubers. The deciding moment came when the fig stopped growing in Europe, for of all fruits, apes love figs the most. Not only do these fruits have especially high fructose content, but fig trees can provide fruit all year around, because fig wasps pollinate the fig throughout the year. Whether it was the loss of the fig or the loss of the wasp that came first, we do not know, but since neither could live without the other, they both disappeared together.

The loss of the fig led to weeks or months in any given year when fruit was unavailable. During this time, the apes were forced to forage for food to avoid starvation. As the weather continued to cool, seasonal starvations worsened, and the isolated colonies of apes slowly disappeared. By 8 to 10 million years ago, the last ape in Europe had perished. These apes were not alone in failing to adjust to the shift in climate: approximately 30 percent of all species died during this time.

This may seem a sad tale, one in which the European ape species became a dead branch in our evolutionary tree. However, anthropologists Peter Andrews from the Natural History Museum in London and David Begun from the University of Toronto separately found fossil evidence that not all of the prehistoric European apes went extinct. Some appear to have survived long enough to successfully return to Africa, where they later evolved into the African apes, as well as you and me, while others journeyed to South Asia where they became the orangutans.

This story turns out to be important because humans and all great apes carry a mutation that results in our species having higher uric acid levels than other mammals. You may recall that uric acid is produced during fructose metabolism and that it has a role in driving the survival switch by causing oxidative stress to the body's energy factories. That all great apes and humans have the same mutation means it came from a common ancestor, raising the possibility that the mutation may have originated in the starving European apes. To investigate this idea, our collaborator, evolutionary biologist Eric Gaucher, used molecular biology to trace the mutation back in time to when it first arose. He calculated that the gene had undergone a stepwise reduction in activity over millions of years, but that it had been completely silenced around 15 million years ago, right at the height of the apes' starvation.

To better understand the role of the mutation, I flew to London to meet Peter Andrews, who, in addition to his discovery of the aforementioned fossil evidence, is a world expert on Miocene apes. Peter agreed that a mutation that enhanced fat formation from fruit could have been lifesaving. He also explained that the survival pressures during that period were weaker in Africa than in Europe, as the temperatures in Africa remained warm enough that, although the apes' habitats contracted, fruit remained available year-round. Therefore, the mutation would have had the most impact if it had occurred in Europe or Asia Minor, where the apes were under the greatest threat of extinction.

The genetic mutation that affected uric acid levels did so by inactivating an enzyme called **uricase**, which normally breaks down uric acid so that levels in the blood remain low. When uricase is absent, the rise in uric acid in response to fructose is heightened. In theory, a higher uric acid level would result in greater oxidative stress to the energy factories, and therefore a greater activation of the survival switch and a higher production of fat for the same amount of fructose. In other words, it would have a similar effect as the loss of our ability to make vitamin C.

We decided to test this hypothesis. First, to understand the impact of a higher uric acid level on fructose metabolism, my collaborator Gaby Sanchez-Lozada blocked the uricase enzyme in laboratory rats using an inhibitor. When she did this, the rats' uric acid level rose. She then fed the same amount of fructose to both the normal rats and the rats whose uricase was inhibited. The striking finding was that the rats with inhibited uricase responded to the fructose with a higher uric acid level and greater oxidative stress compared to the normal rats, and this was associated with higher blood pressure, blood triglycerides, and blood glucose levels, and more fat accumulation in the liver. They also tended to gain more weight, although the amount was not statistically significant, likely because the study only lasted eight weeks.

Next, we collaborated with Eric Gaucher, who resurrected the ancient uricase gene using state-of-the-art molecular biologic techniques. When cultured human liver cells that included this gene were exposed to fructose, some uric acid and fat were made. However, when we did the same to normal human liver cells, in which the uricase gene was missing, the liver cells made more uric acid and twice as much fat for the same amount of fructose. In other words, the presence of the ancient uricase gene in the liver still allowed it to make fat from fructose, but when this uricase was silenced by a mutation, the liver could make much more fat in response to the same amount of fructose.

These studies suggest that we narrowly survived extinction not once but twice in our past thanks to mutations that made us more sensitive to the effects of fructose than many other animals and therefore helped us store fat more effectively. This gave us a decisive advantage when it came to surviving difficult periods when food was not readily available. However, this increased sensitivity is a double-edged sword.

We narrowly survived extinction not once but twice thanks to mutations that made us more sensitive to the effects of fructose.

THRIFTY GENES AND THE RISE OF OBESITY

Sixty years ago, a geneticist named James Neel proposed a hypothesis for why so many people in the Western world were becoming obese and contracting diabetes. His theory came from studying indigenous cultures in which diabetes was infrequent. He suggested that, in the past, at times when famines or other disasters threatened our extinction, we may have acquired mutations that enhanced our survival during these harsh times—such as an improved ability to store fat. And although these mutations would have aided survival during times when food was scarce, in settings where food was easily available, these mutations might backfire and increase the risk for obesity and diabetes.

This "**thrifty gene**" hypothesis had been challenged by many scientists, because no new genes driving obesity have been identified, and also because some people interpret the hypothesis to mean that if we all carry these new genes, then we should all be obese and diabetic. However, our work supports it. Though our studies suggest we did not gain two new genes, but rather lost two old genes, the concept is the same. So how could we test whether this might be true? What sets of experiments could be done?

I thought about the uric acid mutation first. Our hypothesis did not propose that the mutation in uric acid made the Miocene apes fat; rather, we thought it likely protected them from starvation. Perhaps, in most contexts, the uric acid mutation only raised uric acid levels high enough to maintain fat stores, and it required a Western diet of foods rich in fructose to take uric acid to levels that caused frank obesity. Most adults with obesity have blood uric acid levels of 6 mg/dL or more, versus the 4 to 5 mg/dL found in most lean individuals.

Since the mutation occurred in an ancestor of both humans and the great apes, I realized that if I measured the uric acid levels in gorillas or chimpanzees, whose evolutionary branch diverged after the mutation occurred, I could get a better idea of the impact of the mutation on uric acid levels prior to the introduction of a Western diet. So I visited the San Diego Zoo, and met up with Bruce Rideout, who runs a research laboratory there. Together we measured the uric acid levels in a wide range of monkeys and apes. What we found was that the uric acid levels were low (1–2 mg/dL) in primates that expressed the uricase gene, but were modestly higher in the great apes that lacked it (3–4 mg/dL).

I also wanted to measure uric acid levels in people who were not on a Western diet. In my reading of the work of James Neel, I learned he had gone on an expedition to the jungles of the Amazon, where he had studied a group of hunter-gatherers known as the Yanomami. The Yanomami's diet consisted of plants such as plantains and tubers, and wild game. Neel and his colleague William Oliver reported that, despite living stressful lives that included local wars, the Yanomami tended to have low or normal blood pressure and no obesity or diabetes.

I decided this would be a great group to study, and was able to reach Bill Oliver and get blood samples from that original expedition. When we tested them, we found that the Yanomami's uric acid levels were around 3 mg/dL, while the members of Neel's expedition (including Neel himself) all had levels of 5 mg/dL or higher. In other words, our theory seemed to be correct: the mutation only raised our uric acid levels a little, from 1–2 mg/dl in primates that still produce uricase to the 3 mg/dl seen in the Yanomami. (The higher levels of uric acid seen in Neel's expedition members, similar to the levels we see today, were likely due to the effects of the Western diet.) This small rise protected us against starvation but was not in itself enough to cause obesity. The uricase mutation might, however, predispose individuals to develop obesity if they ingest a lot of fructose.

The same is true for the mutation that knocked out our ability to make vitamin C: it might predispose us to develop obesity when our diet is high in fructose. Today, our vitamin C levels vary greatly, since they are largely dependent on fruit intake. Many studies have shown that people who are overweight or who have metabolic syndrome tend to have lower blood levels of vitamin C. There are also studies that suggest increasing vitamin C intake reduces the risk for developing metabolic syndrome. In particular, vitamin C dosages of 500 mg daily have been reported to improve blood pressure, reduce blood triglycerides, increase HDL cholesterol (the good cholesterol), and lower BMI in several studies. Interestingly, giving fruit juice does not seem to be as effective as taking vitamin C supplements, which makes sense, as fruit juice is also rich in fructose.

We became especially sensitive to the effects of fructose millions of years ago, but for most of our history, we have been able to stay lean because our exposure to fructose was limited. When did this change? And what can we learn from that history?

THE EARLIEST EVIDENCE OF OBESITY

Originally, these lifesaving mutations involving our uric acid and vitamin C levels did not make us fat. The fructose we ate mainly came from fruit and honey, which were available only seasonally, and obesity was rare.

How can I confidently make such statements about humans who lived so long ago? Because of telltale signs found in ancient skeletons.

One of the best signs of exposure to fructose is the presence of dental cavities. Cavities are caused by specific bacteria that reside in the mouth and live off the fructose we eat, and cause dental decay and gum disease by releasing acids and other substances that damage teeth and tissues. Thus, the presence of cavities in ancient teeth almost always means that their owner ingested fructose. While occasional cavities could just reflect the intermittent eating of fruit, a high frequency of cavities usually indicates heavy fructose exposure.*

Skeletons also can give us clues about the presence of obesity. When we are overweight or obese, it can put strain on our back, hardening the ligaments and tendons where they attach to the spine, fusing vertebrae, and causing an unusual bone formation. A classic site for this formation in people with obesity is along the spine's right side. This unusual growth has a name: DISH, which stands for "diffuse idiopathic skeletal hyperostosis." Thus, if a skeleton has DISH and a lot of dental cavities, it would strongly suggest that the individual had a history of heavy fructose ingestion and obesity.

For much of history, dental cavities and DISH seem to have been rare. This suggests that heavy fructose consumption and obesity were also uncommon. As we mentioned in chapter one, fertility figurines from the end of the Upper Paleolithic period in Europe suggest some obesity may have occurred during that period, and skeletons dating to the same time show a doubling of dental cavities, but in general, in the Paleolithic period, obesity was likely rare.

Leaping forward in time, there is some evidence of obesity and diabetes in Ancient Egypt around four thousand years ago, possibly linked with honey intake. Honey was especially valued by the Egyptians. It was used as salve for wounds, for mummification, and especially in foods and drinks such as honey

---

* Today, the fluoride added to toothpaste and drinking water kills the bacteria and prevents cavities, so our increased fructose consumption isn't reflected in our teeth in the same way.

cakes and honey-based beer. It was valued like gold and silver, and was often collected as a type of tax or taken as a spoil of war. Thutmose III, for example, collected over 470 jars of honey when he invaded Canaan (today's Israel and Palestine), the "land of milk and honey."

It is not surprising, then, that studies of mummies have documented dental cavities, DISH, and excessive skin folds consistent with obesity among royalty and some of the wealthy. One of the more famous examples was of Hatshepsut, one of the first female pharaohs, who reigned for over twenty years in the fifteenth century BC. Her mummy was found with severe tooth decay, and with evidence she was both obese and diabetic.

While obesity was present in our past, as among the wealthy in Egypt, it was nowhere near as frequent as it is today. To get at the real root of today's obesity epidemic, we have to look at the introduction and spread of one of the greatest discoveries of all time, a white substance that has dominated history as one of the most desired of all foods: table sugar.

THE RISE OF SUGAR

It is to the banks of the Ganges River in India approximately 2,500 years ago that the very beginnings of the obesity epidemic can be traced. There, local farmers discovered that the sugarcane growing along the Ganges provided a sweet liquid once its reeds were boiled and crushed. The Indian physician Sushruta noted that many who drank it frequently developed obesity and diabetes, but its sweetness was too alluring for them to stop. Reports of this delightful substance were brought back to Persia from the exploits of Darius, and also to Greece by soldiers from Alexander the Great's campaign.

Soon thereafter, the art of creating crystalline sugar was developed, and by the Middle Ages sugar had been brought to China, Persia, and Egypt, followed by Cyprus and northern Africa, where the climate allowed sugarcane to be grown. However, very little sugar reached Europe. Moses Maimonides, a twelfth-century Jewish physician, noted that while there was an absence of diabetes in Spain, when he moved to Egypt he saw more than twenty cases. He did not understand why. In retrospect, we do: sugar had not yet reached Spain.

Reports of this food, which tasted better than honey and looked "like snow or white salt," came to Europe in the twelfth and thirteenth centuries with Crusaders returning from the Holy Land. One such Crusader was King Edward I of England, who fell in love with sugar. At the time sugar was extremely expensive and hard to get. But the Republic of Venice had begun to import it from Egypt, Cyprus, and southern Arabia, and Edward liked it so much that, despite its cost, he bought 1,877 pounds of sugar for his household in 1287 and more than thrice that the following year.

The period's royalty were not alone in their obsession. Religious leaders also loved sugar and became fat. St. Thomas Aquinas (1225–1274) liked sugar so much that he declared it a medicine to rationalize ingesting it while fasting. Pope Leo X (1475–1521) loved sugar so much that he was once given life-sized statues of his cardinals made from sugar; he became known as Pope Leo the Fat.

While the wealthy could afford sugar, it remained much too costly for the average person for many years. In the fourteenth century, for example, one pound of sugar cost the equivalent of twenty-eight pounds of cheese or thirty-four dozen eggs.

The economics of sugar changed, however, after sugarcane was introduced to the Americas. By the 1600s, England controlled much of the sugar coming from America, resulting in the infamous "triangle trade," in which sugar was imported to England; the revenues from sugar sales were spent to manufacture gunpowder, lead, and salt, which were traded for slaves in Africa; and enslaved Africans were sent to the Americas to work the sugar and cotton plantations.

Most of the sugar from the Americas was imported to England; very little was exported elsewhere. Soon, sugar houses were arising throughout London, and sugar was being added to coffee, tea, and alcohol. Popular sugar-based drinks included rum, which was distilled from sugarcane, and "sack and sugar." Sack was wine, to which spirits from grapes, sugarcane, or sugar beets were added; crystallized sugar was then added on top. (Sir John Falstaff, a character in several of Shakespeare's plays often portrayed as fat, was a heavy drinker whose nickname was Sack and Sugar, for the drink.) Other favored drinks included hippocras (a wine to which cinnamon, nutmeg, and sugar were added) and punch (in which sugar was added to a combination of wine, brandy, and rum).

Although England continued to dominate sugar imports for the next several hundred years, exporting less and less to the rest of Europe, Holland was also a major player in Europe's sugar trade. By the mid-1600s it was importing sugar from Suriname in South America, as well as from Java and other islands in the East Indies. Both Amsterdam and Antwerp established many sugar refineries, and supplied nearly half of the refined sugar to Europe at that time.

Not surprisingly, it was in these two countries, Holland and England, where obesity first began to rise. As early as 1685, the Dutch physician Steven Blankaart counseled that sugar had played a role in the rapid rise of dental cavities, obesity, and gout (as mentioned, arthritis triggered by uric acid, often resulting from high sugar intake) observed in Holland. Hermann Boerhaave, another famous Dutch physician, wrote about a patient who was so large that he had to use a sash tied around his neck to hold up his belly, and have a section of his dinner table cut out to allow him to sit close enough to reach his food.

By the end of the seventeenth century, the Dutch Golden Age had ended, and their importation of sugar was severely curtailed when England began seizing their ships during the Anglo–Dutch Wars. In contrast, per capita sugar consumption in England continued to rise, from approximately 4 pounds per year in 1700 to 18 pounds in 1800. English grocer Daniel Lambert reached a then-world-record weight of 732 pounds; he wore a "waistcoat that easily could enclose 7 persons of ordinary size." By early 1800, the British physician William Wadd lamented, "For every fat person in France or Spain, there are a hundred in England."

France, however, was not to be outdone. The hoarding of sugar by the British, coupled with the British blockade of ships bringing sugar from the East and West Indies to mainland Europe during the Napoleonic Wars, led Napoleon to search for other ways to get sugar. He found it in the sugar beet. German chemist Andreas Marggraf had successfully developed a method for extracting sugar from sugar beets back in 1747, but their first use for sugar production did not occur until the beginning of the 1800s. Between 1811 and 1815, Napoleon built forty sugar beet factories in France. Soon France, as well as other European countries, were producing enough sugar to supply most of the European continent. The timing was fortuitous: with the birth of the United States, Americans gained more control of the cane sugar trade and were able to keep more sugar for their own citizens.

SUGAR CONSUMED PER CAPITA

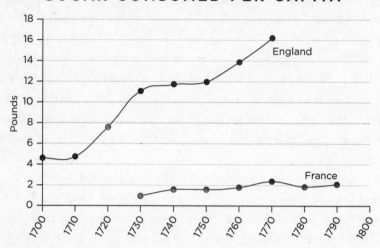

During the eighteenth century, much more sugar was consumed in England than in the rest of Europe (exemplified here by France), and it was in England where the obesity epidemic took hold. (Adapted from Social Science History *14: 95–115.)*

With these new sources, sugar, which had been expensive everywhere except England, started to become affordable. And sugar intake continued to rise around the world. By 1900, per capita sugar consumption had increased in England to about ninety pounds a person per year—an approximate fivefold increase in a single century.

THE TIPPING POINT, AND THE RISE OF OBESITY AND DIABETES IN THE TWENTIETH CENTURY

In the introduction, I suggested that the tipping point in the history of obesity, the time when it suddenly began to increase in the population (along with other epidemics such as diabetes and heart disease), came around the time of the 1893 Chicago World's Fair. Knowing what we know now, we see the emergence of these epidemics in a new light. The main reason was not, I'd argue, the impact of technological advances. It is true that such advances led to rapid industrialization and mass production of goods, reducing the demand for strenuous labor, and that improvements in automobiles, trains, and other types of transportation made it possible to stock stores with foods from distant markets so that there was always plenty to eat.

Nevertheless, the real reason for the emergence of these epidemics, I believe, is the fact that sugar was becoming both more affordable and more available, allowing intake to increase. In 1800, sugar intake in England amounted to only eighteen pounds per person per year, in part because sugar was heavily taxed. With both increased sugar production and progressive reductions in the sugar tax, the consumption of sugar increased. Once Prime Minister William Gladstone finally ended the sugar tax in 1874, sugar consumption increased from around fifty pounds per year to, by the time of the Chicago Fair, approximately ninety pounds per year. The US initially lagged slightly behind, with an intake of about sixty pounds per year in 1893, but this increased to eighty-five pounds

ADDED SUGAR INTAKE IN THE US AND UK

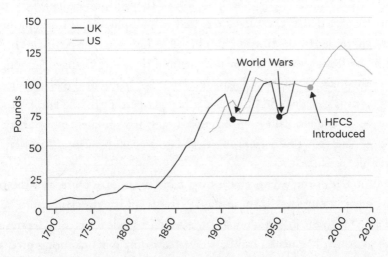

The rise in sugar (sucrose) consumption in pounds per person per year in the United Kingdom (1700-1930) and the United States (1890-2020). Sugar consumption in the United Kingdom accelerated as the sugar tax was reduced, while sugar consumption fell during the world wars. Beginning in 1975, HFCS is included in total sugar intake. (Adapted from Noël Deer, The History of Sugar; Nature 239: 197-199; Arch Int Medicine 1924; 34: 585-630; United States Census Bureau.)

per year by the beginning of World War I. Furthermore, soft drinks such as Coca-Cola, Dr Pepper, and Pepsi Cola were introduced during this time, and soda fountains were becoming popular. This rise in sugar intake in the twentieth century was paralleled by a rise in both obesity and diabetes.

The real reason for the emergence of the obesity and diabetes epidemics is that sugar was becoming both more affordable and more available, allowing intake to increase.

The evidence that it is sugar that is driving obesity is extensive. Numerous studies have shown that the introduction of sugar into a community is almost inevitably followed by a rise in obesity and diabetes. This has been observed throughout the world, often in remote or isolated populations. For example, obesity and diabetes rapidly increased among the Polynesians, the Maori, the Tiwi, and Native Americans with the introduction of sugar.

On Nauru, a small island in the Pacific, residents lived primarily on fish, breadfruit, and coconuts. Then, in the early 1900s, Europeans discovered that the island was rich in phosphates, and mining began, largely controlled by the British Phosphate Commission. The Nauruans became wealthy by leasing their land for mining, and their diet changed. Among the foods brought to Nauru was sugar, and by 1925, many of the Nauruans were eating as much as a pound of sugar per day per person. By the late 1920s, the first cases of diabetes had been diagnosed, and the prevalence of obesity and diabetes increased rapidly from there. Today, over 90 percent of Nauruans are overweight or obese.

For much of the twentieth century, table sugar, or sucrose, was the main added sugar in our diet. Then, in the 1970s, use of fructose-containing sugars accelerated with the invention of a new sweetener made from corn. Corn sugar, which is primarily glucose, can be converted in the manufacturing process to fructose, the sweeter of these two sugars. This allows the mixing of glucose and fructose to make high-fructose corn syrup. While sucrose is always an equal ratio of fructose to glucose because the two molecules are bonded together, HFCS can vary in its fructose-to-glucose ratio. Its 55:45 ratio of fructose to glucose—or even higher, 65:35—creates an even sweeter taste that many people prefer to standard table sugar. HFCS became a popular additive in processed foods. Because it is liquid, and therefore easy to mix, food manufacturers were able to add it to foods that normally contained no or minimal sucrose. Sucrose also tends to crystallize in foods during prolonged storage, while HFCS does not. Although it was originally intended to replace sucrose in foods, sucrose has continued to be used as well, with the consequence that total intake of these two added sugars rose precipitously in the late 1970s, rising from a per-person intake of about 95 pounds per year in 1970 to nearly 130 pounds per year in 2000. And with that rise came a further increase in obesity and diabetes.

THE ECONOMICS OF SUGAR, AND RISK OF OBESITY AND DIABETES

Over the centuries, the risk for obesity and diabetes has tracked with sugar intake. Thus, researchers have been able to use the relative cost of sugar to predict who is at greatest risk. A clear example is in Ceylon (now part of Sri Lanka) in the early 1800s, where diabetes was observed primarily among the poor, who, unlike the wealthy in Ceylon, ate a lot of palm sugar as well as fructose-heavy foods like plantain, jackfruit, and yams.

In the early 1900s, sugar was still relatively expensive in the United States, and a study from New York City found obesity and diabetes were rare among Black Americans but much more common among the wealthy. Today, sugar and HFCS have become inexpensive, and the epidemiology has reversed. It is the disadvantaged—minority populations and the poor—that suffer the most from obesity and diabetes, as it is these groups that are, largely for economic reasons, consuming the most added sugars. The rates of obesity and diabetes are not intrinsically higher in the minority populations, but rather reflect the economics of sugar.

CLINICAL EVIDENCE THAT ADDED SUGARS ARE DRIVING THE OBESITY AND DIABETES EPIDEMICS

Today, sucrose and high-fructose corn syrup account for 15 to 20 percent of the total calories we take in, and some people are getting 25 percent or more of their calories from these two added sugars. Both sucrose and HFCS contain fructose, so a consequence of the increased intake of both sugars is that we are also increasing our fructose intake. Today, most of our fructose comes not from fruits and honey but from sucrose and HFCS. Therefore, intake of these sugars can be viewed as a surrogate for fructose intake.

The epidemiology is straightforward. As we've seen, the rise in sucrose and HFCS parallels the rise in obesity and diabetes. The introduction of these sugars into a population is followed by a rise in obesity and diabetes. And within populations, individuals who consume the most added sugar tend to have the highest risk of developing these conditions. This is especially true when you look at soft drink intake.

The consumption of sucrose and HFCS peaked around 2000, and has been slowly decreasing since. Beginning in 2005, soft drink consumption also began to fall (although this has been partially made up for by a rise in "energy drinks" high in sugar or HFCS). As expected, this has been accompanied by evidence of a slowdown in the obesity and diabetes epidemics; for the first time, the number of new cases of diabetes is decreasing. Nevertheless, overall intake of sucrose and HFCS remains high, especially among adolescents and minority populations, and the prevalence of obesity and diabetes remains high as well.

While the epidemiology strongly implicates sucrose and HFCS in these epidemics, association does not equal causality. Teasing out the reason for the association between added sugar and obesity and diabetes is where clinical studies come in. You can give fructose, sucrose, or HFCS to individuals, and determine what happens.

Some of the best evidence for a causal role of fructose in metabolic syndrome comes from a ten-week study of overweight individuals performed by Kimber Stanhope and Peter Havel from the University of California, Davis, which we touched on in chapter three. In this study, each day individuals had to drink water to which either fructose or glucose had been added. The individuals who drank fructose showed weight gain, a decrease in resting metabolism, abdominal fat accumulation, an elevation in blood triglycerides, the development of insulin resistance, a rise in inflammatory markers and uric acid in the blood, and worsened liver function. In contrast, individuals who were given glucose, while they showed similar weight gain, had significantly fewer metabolic changes. This study therefore suggested that there was something distinct about fructose and its ability to induce features of metabolic syndrome.

We also performed a similar study with clinician Enrique Perez-Pozo in which we provided overweight men with a daily fructose drink for two weeks. The drink, which was equivalent to four to five 20-ounce soft drinks, was provided in two 1-liter bottles that the subjects drank from throughout the day. Admittedly, this is more fructose than the typical person drinks (though not too different from what some adolescents and young adults are consuming on a daily basis, incredibly). However, we were interested in whether high doses of fructose given for a short period (two weeks) might reproduce metabolic effects that would typically take months or years.

After two weeks of drinking the fructose solution, these men showed significant elevations in their blood pressure, increased fats in their blood, and worsening insulin resistance. The effects were so significant that, by the end of the study, fully 25 percent of the men met the definition of having metabolic syndrome when previously they had not. To observe these changes occurring so rapidly was disquieting, and I do not believe that we could ever in good conscience do such a study again. Fortunately, once the fructose was stopped, these effects reversed over the next several weeks.

In real life, most people do not drink fructose alone, but rather drink fructose and glucose together either as sucrose or HFCS, and often in the form of soft drinks. It is therefore important to look at studies evaluating the effects of soft drinks on our metabolic health.

One such study was conducted by Maria Maersk and her colleagues from Aarhus University Hospital in Denmark. They randomized overweight subjects into four groups, each of which was assigned to ingest a liter a day of either soft drinks, diet soft drinks, milk, or water for six months. Participants were otherwise allowed to drink their desired amount of water, tea, coffee, or alcohol. After six months, extensive testing was done, including measuring the fat mass in various organs. The findings were striking: the individuals in the soft drinks group showed a significant increase in abdominal fat, liver fat, and both blood triglycerides and total cholesterol. They also had higher blood pressure than the groups that drank milk and diet soft drinks (though not, oddly, water). This study suggests that added sugars likely have a role in causing metabolic syndrome in humans.

Another way to look at the metabolic role of fructose is by observing the effects of restricting fructose in the diet. To study this, Robert Lustig and Jean-Marc Schwarz from the University of California, San Francisco performed a study in which adolescents reduced their intake of fructose-containing sugars from 28 to 10 percent, while substituting in starch so that their total caloric intake remained the same. After nine days, the teens showed a significant decrease in weight, body fat, blood triglycerides, LDL cholesterol (the bad cholesterol), and diastolic blood pressure, as well as improved insulin resistance.

Miriam Vos, a pediatrician at Emory University in Atlanta, performed a study in which adolescent boys with documented fatty liver were randomly assigned to eat either a diet low in added sugars or a regular diet for eight weeks. The subjects who were on the low-added-sugar diet showed a remarkable improvement in the severity of their fatty liver.

Sucrose and HFCS, both of which contain fructose, are playing a major role in the obesity epidemic and our worsening metabolic health, and specific studies of fructose alone suggest that fructose, rather than glucose, is the main sugar responsible. The trial is over. The verdict is in. Fructose is guilty (though it is we who are sentenced). There is, however, a twist—a big surprise that is just around the corner.

CHAPTER 5

An Unpleasant Surprise: It's Not Just Fructose

A s our research progressed, I became convinced that fructose intake was the major cause of the metabolic syndrome and obesity, and that the way to prevent the two was to reduce fructose intake. I started recommending a low-fructose diet to friends, neighbors, and patients as the first step to treating obesity. One of the first people to whom I prescribed this diet was the son of one of my research associates, who had been diagnosed with an enlarged fatty liver. Within just a few months of cutting out soft drinks, the fat in his liver had melted away and his liver was back to its normal size.

Based on early success, I became convinced that the reason low-carbohydrate diets are so effective is that they restrict fructose consumption. I thought it wasn't important to reduce foods that are high in starch (such as rice and potatoes) because they are not high in fructose, although they are high in glucose. It seemed possible to design a diet as effective as a low-carb diet in which one could still eat carbohydrates, so long as those carbohydrates did not contain fructose. In 2008, I wrote a book, *The Sugar Fix*, that was one of the first books to identify fructose as the culprit of the obesity epidemic, and in it I introduced a low-fructose diet as the solution to the obesity epidemic. I was on a roll!

But while many people told me my diet was effective, others on it failed to lose much weight. I had a particularly troubling interview with Jimmy Moore, an entertaining and gracious personality who produces a podcast called *Livin' La Vida Low-Carb*. Jimmy had lost 180 pounds by following a low-carb diet, and he told me that he ended up having to restrict all carbohydrates to lose weight. I was bothered by this observation; I too had noticed how certain foods, such as bread, seemed to be fattening even when they were low in fructose.

I also knew that fructose could not explain how some animals, such as the whale and the camel, become obese. After all, these animals do not have much access to foods rich in fructose, such as fruit and honey. It seemed to me that we were missing something major. Perhaps fructose was only part of the story. Or perhaps, just perhaps, there was a source of fructose that I had not yet considered.

A SECRET SOURCE OF FRUCTOSE

The great assumption that we, as well as the rest of the world, were making was that the only fructose that mattered when it came to health and disease was the fructose we consume. Our big discovery was that there is *another* major source of fructose that can trigger the survival switch, and thus cause obesity and metabolic syndrome: the fructose that *our bodies make*.

Scientists have known for decades that the body can make fructose. A special biological process known as the **polyol pathway** first converts glucose to a substance known as **sorbitol**,* then further converts the sorbitol to fructose. But while the polyol pathway is well known, it is generally thought to be minimally active in most people, such that it produced an inconsequential amount of fructose.

The polyol pathway plays a role in early pregnancy, as well as in the kidney, where it helps in the reabsorption of water in response to dehydration. But it is best known for its activation in diabetes, where high blood-glucose levels

---

* You may recognize sorbitol as an artificial sweetener that is often added to "sugar-free" syrups. Unfortunately, sorbitol is turned into sugar—fructose—in the body.

trigger the production of sorbitol and fructose. There is even some evidence that the sorbitol generated in diabetes can contribute to some of the medical complications associated with the disease, such as cataracts and nerve damage. However, there was little concern in the literature about the fructose made by the same pathway.

This would all change when molecular biologist Miguel Lanaspa* joined my laboratory in 2010. By coincidence, Miguel had studied the polyol pathway with his previous mentor. Early on, he and I had several discussions about whether the fructose made from the polyol pathway might play a role in certain diabetes complications, such as weight gain, worsening insulin resistance, fatty liver, and kidney disease—a fertile topic for study.

One day I shared with Miguel my concerns about the evidence that one could develop obesity and metabolic syndrome from carbohydrates even if they did not contain fructose. Miguel then proposed a very exciting possibility: What if eating certain carbohydrates released so much glucose following digestion that it mimicked the diabetic state, activating the polyol pathway and generating fructose? When glucose is absorbed, it must first pass through the liver, where much of it is metabolized before it reaches the bloodstream. Therefore, the liver sees the highest glucose concentrations and is the site where the most fructose would be produced. As we learned previously, the liver is also the critical organ where fructose metabolism drives the survival switch. If these high levels of glucose led to the production of sufficient fructose, it might trigger the survival switch without one having to ingest fructose at all—thus explaining why Jimmy Moore had to reduce all carbohydrates in order to lose weight.

It was a great hypothesis, but of course we needed to test it. We decided to do so by adding pure glucose to the drinking water of laboratory mice. This ensured high concentrations of glucose in the gut and therefore high concentrations of glucose reaching the liver and then the bloodstream beyond. The first thing we noted was how much the animals liked to drink glucose; they drank as much or more water containing glucose as mice offered water containing the same concentrations of sucrose, HFCS, or fructose. They also ate more food,

---

* I have mentioned Miguel several times already, as he has become one of my major long-term collaborators and has had a profound impact on our research. I began as his mentor, but gradually we became equals in our studies to dissect the role of fructose in health and disease.

and started becoming fat and insulin resistant. For someone like me who had previously believed that fructose was the only carbohydrate that could cause metabolic syndrome, the experiment was off to a depressing start.

Over the next few months, the mice became super fat—so rotund that they waddled when they walked. They also developed insulin resistance and fatty liver. The moment of truth came at the end of the experiment, when we found very high levels of fructose in their livers even though they had been eating no fructose at all. We also found evidence that the polyol pathway was turned on, as shown by high levels of one of the enzymes involved. Miguel was right!

To understand how the fructose being produced affected the development of obesity and metabolic syndrome, we also gave glucose to mice that had been genetically altered such that they could not metabolize fructose. These mice could metabolize glucose normally, and drank the same amount of glucose as the original mice. But that is where the similarities ended. Unlike the original mice that had been given glucose, these special mice developed much less obesity and were almost completely protected from developing fatty liver and insulin resistance.

We also performed another study, this time using mice that lacked the ability to *make* fructose, due to removal of a gene coding for one of the key enzymes in the polyol pathway. These mice, too, still liked glucose, but were similarly protected from developing obesity and metabolic syndrome.

It was a major breakthrough, simultaneously exhilarating and depressing. It is not just the fructose we eat that causes obesity; it is the fructose we make. What is more, glucose, a major component of the carbohydrates in our diet, could be converted to fructose in our body. Yes, there was a little evidence that glucose itself could cause some obesity, for the animals that received glucose but whose fructose production or metabolism was blocked still gained some weight compared to mice on a normal diet. However, much of the weight gain, and almost all of the insulin resistance and fatty liver, that follows high intake of glucose appears due to the fructose that the body makes from that glucose.

> *It is not just the fructose we eat that causes obesity; it is the fructose we make.*

HIGH-GLYCEMIC CARBOHYDRATES AS A MEANS OF ACTIVATING THE SURVIVAL SWITCH

If glucose causes obesity and metabolic syndrome by being converted to fructose, then it raises the question of whether other carbohydrates could do the same. One would not expect all carbohydrates to be equivalent in their ability to generate fructose, however. Because the polyol pathway is activated by high glucose levels, only carbohydrates that tend to break down to glucose quickly and easily would trigger the process.

The difference in the ability of carbohydrates to raise blood glucose is reflected in a measurement called the **glycemic index**. A food's glycemic index is a numeric value representing its ability to increase blood glucose two hours after a meal. Pure glucose has a value of 100, and foods that do not raise blood glucose at all have a value of 0. Foods that release glucose rapidly after digestion—foods with a glycemic index of 70 or higher—are called **high-glycemic foods**.* Some of the more common high-glycemic foods include breads (especially white bread), rice (especially white rice), potatoes (both regular and sweet), cereals, chips, and crackers.

You have probably heard the term "high-glycemic foods" before, as their association with obesity and metabolic syndrome is widely accepted and has been for decades. (It is this type of carbohydrate that most low-carb diets aim to reduce.) Our studies suggest that the way these foods might cause obesity is by stimulating the production of fructose. However, this viewpoint differs from what has been proposed in the literature. Most experts have suggested that the way high-glycemic carbohydrates cause obesity is by stimulating the release of insulin, which enhances the uptake of glucose into various tissues. This extra glucose is then made into energy (ATP) or stored as glycogen or fat, and over time, obesity results. Indeed, many people with obesity have chronically high insulin levels.

The insulin hypothesis has been suggested as the reason why soft drinks cause obesity and metabolic syndrome. Soft drinks have a high glycemic index because they contain sucrose or HFCS, both of which contain glucose in

---

* "Glycemia" is a medical term that refers to the concentration of glucose in the blood.

addition to fructose. The ingestion of fructose itself does not raise blood glucose very much because fructose has a low glycemic index, only about 19, and fructose also does not directly increase insulin levels; this means the rapid rise in glucose and insulin after consuming a soft drink is primarily from the glucose in the soft drink and not the fructose. So, according to the classical view of the insulin hypothesis, it must be the glucose component of soft drinks that leads to obesity.

Miguel and I realized we could do an experiment that would prove whether glucose or fructose was responsible. We gave drinking water spiked with HFCS to both normal mice and mice that could not metabolize fructose. (Because the mice that could not metabolize fructose did not like HFCS as much as normal mice, we had to provide water with higher concentrations of HFCS to these mice to assure equivalent intake.) As expected, the normal mice that were given soft drinks became fat and developed all of the features of metabolic syndrome. In contrast, the mice that could not metabolize fructose gained minimal weight and remained healthy despite ingesting the same amount of HFCS. In particular, they did not develop insulin resistance or fatty liver—despite consuming a large amount of glucose from the HFCS.

Thus, the reason soft drinks cause obesity is because of fructose—likely from both that present in the drink and that generated from the glucose soft drinks contain. While fructose does not itself stimulate insulin, when fructose is metabolized, it activates the survival switch, which over time causes the development of insulin resistance. This then results in chronic elevations of both glucose and insulin. So the observation remains the same: drinking high-glycemic soft drinks leads to high glucose and insulin levels and obesity, and high-glycemic carbohydrates (i.e., the glucose) play a role in causing metabolic syndrome. However, these conditions do not arise from the direct stimulation of insulin by glucose, but rather because some of the glucose is being converted to fructose. The cause of metabolic syndrome is fructose.

The reason carbohydrates cause obesity and metabolic syndrome is primarily due to their ability to stimulate fructose production.

WHY IS BREAD FATTENING? BLAME
THE BIRTH OF CIVILIZATION

Remember Jim Neel's theory of thrifty genes, and how two mutations in our distant past that helped us survive when food was scarce now increase our risk for obesity? There may be yet a third "thrifty gene" playing a role in our obesity epidemic.

The first agricultural communities developed around the Black Sea and in the Middle East approximately 10,000 to 12,000 years ago. There, archaeological evidence suggests that the first domesticated crop may have been the fig (one of the richest food sources of fructose), and that barley and wheat were introduced soon afterward. Eating these latter foods was difficult for many early farmers, as their high starch content made them difficult to digest. Humans back then produced only small amounts of **amylase**,* the main enzyme that breaks down starch into glucose, in their saliva. However, around that time, a genetic mutation occurred that resulted in us being able to make double or triple the amount—or even more—of this enzyme, and these higher concentrations made breaking down starch much easier and quicker. This increase in amylase also meant more glucose was released in the mouth, where it triggered the sweet taste buds on the tongue and made high-starch content foods taste better.

Today, the majority of individuals in agricultural communities (about 70 percent) have high concentrations of amylase in their saliva due to this mutation, as compared to only a minority of hunter-gatherers (about 30 percent). Theoretically, individuals with higher concentrations of amylase would be at greater risk for developing obesity from high-glycemic carbohydrates, but this is not yet proven, and more studies are needed.

---

* Amylase is the reason placing a cracker in your mouth results in a sweet taste after a minute; the sweet taste represents the conversion of the starch to glucose.

PRODUCING FRUCTOSE AS A SURVIVAL STRATEGY

The discovery that our bodies can make fructose, and that they can make enough to make us fat, was a great revelation. It was something no one had considered before. And Miguel and I immediately wanted to know more about how the polyol pathway is turned on. Indeed, it dawned on us that other foods we were eating might also be converted to fructose in our body. We realized that we, and the rest of the scientists studying sugar, had only been looking at half of the equation: how much fructose was being eaten. It might be equally as important to understand the factors driving how much fructose we make.

While the best-known way of activating the polyol pathway is elevated blood glucose levels in uncontrolled diabetes, other conditions have also been shown to stimulate fructose production. What struck me was that these were all conditions in which activating the survival switch might be helpful.

For example, the polyol pathway is also activated by dehydration, as when an animal does not have adequate water. This makes sense, as the fat accumulation stimulated by fructose would provide a source of metabolic water. Likewise, the pathway is activated when blood pressure drops, reducing blood flow to our organs and tissues (which can mean they do not get the nutrients they need to function). The generation of fructose helps us hold on to salt, raising blood pressure and improving circulation. Conditions such as a heart attack, in which the blood supply to heart tissue is compromised, or situations where oxygen levels are low, activate the polyol pathway as well. Fructose production in these conditions might be beneficial by suppressing the function of our oxygen-dependent energy factories, thereby reducing oxygen needs. Our group also found the polyol pathway could additionally be stimulated by fructose itself—or rather, by the uric acid generated during fructose's metabolism—which could act as an amplifying system to assist survival.

In other words, the conditions that stimulate our body to produce fructose are the same ones in which it would be desirable to activate the survival switch. This suggests that the polyol pathway—due to its unique ability to produce fructose—is likely used as a backup survival plan when fructose-rich foods cannot be found.

FRUCTOSE IS PRODUCED
IN TIMES OF STRESS

The body makes fructose via the polyol pathway when:

- glucose levels are high (e.g., in uncontrolled diabetes).
- the body is dehydrated.
- blood pressure is low.
- blood supply is impaired (e.g., during heart attack).
- oxygen is low (e.g., at high altitude).
- uric acid levels are high.
- fructose is ingested.

The generation of fructose is therefore a response to stress that aids survival. But let's think back to nature. In nature the best option is not to be caught in a disaster unprepared, but rather to be ready when it happens. This is why animals activate the survival switch before they hibernate or migrate long distances. And if they can do this by eating fruits and honey rich in fructose, could they also do so by triggering fructose production? Might there be foods, for example, that mimic a crisis, such that the body would activate the polyol pathway and generate fructose, to protect us from the winter to come?

The ability to produce our own fructose is a backup survival plan for when fructose-rich foods cannot be found.

SALT: A NONCALORIC SUBSTANCE
THAT CAN MAKE US FAT

There is an interesting observation in nature, which is that many animals, especially hooved mammals, love salt licks. There are places in the wild where the ground is high in minerals and salts, and these natural salt licks are especially attractive to deer, which will travel long distances to find them. Some studies have shown that, although salt licks contain many minerals, it is the salt that animals seek.

The reason deer and other animals love salt licks is not fully understood, for while salt may taste good, it also can make animals thirsty—not a satisfying feeling. However, some studies have found that visiting salt licks is associated with weight gain. For example, a study in the 1970s in New Zealand showed that providing salt dramatically improved the weight of cattle who were grazing primarily on alfalfa. This raised the interesting possibility: Could salt licks be a way to activate the survival switch?

As we know, dehydration stimulates the production of fructose in the body by activating the polyol pathway. Typically, dehydration is associated with not drinking enough water, or with the loss of water, such as from sweating or diarrhea. The amount of water in our blood drops, the concentration of salt in our blood rises, and this rise in concentration results in us becoming thirsty and seeking water. However, we can also "create" dehydration by eating salty foods, as this also increases the salt concentration in our blood and stimulates thirst.

Could animals have learned to crave salt licks because they help create a dehydrated state that stimulates fructose production? Given the relatively poor caloric content of the grasses that deer and similar animals eat, activating the switch would be a valuable way to help them both make and store fat. Furthermore, dehydration could also be an important stimulus for fat storage in other animals, such as the camel and whale in their extreme low-water (in the whale's case, low *fresh*water) environments.

Miguel and I realized that we could test this hypothesis by giving a salty diet to laboratory mice to see if mild dehydration might cause obesity. To do this, we placed laboratory mice on a high-salt diet and compared them with mice on a regular diet. For the first few months, there was no difference in their weight, even though the mice on the high-salt diet ate more. However, after five or six months, the mice on the high-salt diet had become extraordinarily fat compared to mice on a normal-salt diet. They also had most of the features of metabolic syndrome, including fatty liver and prediabetes. As expected for having been on a high-salt diet for months, they showed a rise in blood pressure and some thickening (hypertrophy) of the heart. But most exciting for us, we found high levels of fructose in their livers and brains, despite there being minimal fructose in their diet.

While we were running this experiment, we also gave a high-salt diet to a different group of mice genetically engineered to be unable to metabolize fructose. Despite eating the same amount of salt as the normal high-salt-diet mice, these mice stayed lean and were completely protected from developing fatty liver, insulin resistance, and other features of metabolic syndrome. They also did not show any rise in blood pressure and had minimal thickening of the heart.

In other words, almost all of salt's negative health effects were a consequence of salt stimulating fructose production. Even the well-known effect of salt on blood pressure appears to depend on fructose. Clearly the relationship between salt and sugar is stronger than anticipated.

From a nutrition standpoint, the observation that a high-salt diet can cause obesity may seem surprising. Salt has no calories. However, in our study, the reason a high-salt diet caused obesity was not the salt itself, but rather the high salt concentration in the blood that activated the polyol system. That system converted much of the glucose the mice ate to fructose, which was then metabolized, activating the survival switch.

High-salt diets cause obesity and metabolic syndrome by stimulating fructose production in the body.

Is the observation that salty foods cause obesity in laboratory animals relevant to us? Most of the research on salt and humans focuses on its association with blood pressure and heart disease, but high-salt diets are also associated with obesity and diabetes. Back in the early 1990s, a study was done in which healthy individuals were placed on either a very low-salt diet (0.5 g salt/day) or a high-salt diet (12 g salt/day) for just five days. At the end of five days, the subjects eating the high-salt diet were already showing early signs of insulin resistance. Small epidemiologic studies have also reported that subjects with obesity or metabolic syndrome tend to eat a high-salt diet. And studies from Germany, Finland, and Denmark have reported that both children and adults on a high-salt diet are at increased risk for developing obesity and metabolic syndrome later in life.

In 2018, Masanari Kuwabara, a Japanese cardiologist, conducted a study with our research team that looked at the relationship of salt intake to obesity and metabolic syndrome in a group of adults getting their health care through a hospital program in Japan. Japan is a country where intake of salt is high and intake of sugar is low compared to Western countries such as the United States, and in Kuwabara's study population, the average intake of salt was 11 grams per day. Kuwabara divided the program participants into two groups: those who ate less than 11 grams of salt per day and those who ate more. At the end of five years, those who ate a higher salt diet were at increased risk for developing both diabetes and fatty liver. The risk for obesity was not different, but this is possibly because the follow-up time was too soon for a statistical difference to occur. While higher salt intake also correlated with higher overall calorie intake, those with low calorie intake but high salt intake were still at increased risk for developing fatty liver, and had a stronger tendency to develop diabetes. This study provided additional evidence linking high salt intake with later development of metabolic syndrome and diabetes.

Consistent with the observation that obesity is associated with a high-salt diet, there is also strong evidence that individuals with obesity are chronically dehydrated. Their water intake is often low, the salt concentration in their blood tends to be high, and they are often thirsty. One study, led by nutritionist Jodi Stookey, found that people who are overweight are about 30 percent more likely to be dehydrated (based on the salt concentration in the blood) as their leaner counterparts, while people with obesity are twice as likely to be dehydrated.

People with obesity are ten times as likely to be dehydrated as their leaner counterparts.

One way that dehydration can be assessed is by measuring the blood level of the hormone **vasopressin**. Vasopressin's main job is to protect animals from dehydration by helping the body hold on to water, and the main way it works is by helping the kidneys reabsorb water from urine. Some studies suggest it may also reduce loss of water from the lungs.* Not surprisingly, desert mammals—for whom it is particularly important to conserve water—have very high vasopressin levels.

Blood vasopressin is also high in people who are overweight or obese. Studies led by nutritionists Sofia Enhörning and Olle Melander from Sweden that

---

* Every time we breathe out, we lose a little water vapor in addition to ridding ourselves of carbon dioxide.

measured vasopressin's precursor, copeptin, have found not only that vasopressin levels are high in subjects with obesity and metabolic syndrome, but that, if a lean person has a high level of copeptin, they are at increased risk for developing obesity and diabetes in the future.

Our detective work is paying off. Salt, and specifically its ability to create a mild state of dehydration, appears to be another way to trigger the survival switch. Eating fruits and honey rich in fructose creates a false sense of starvation that encourages fat production, allowing animals to prepare for hibernation by increasing their stores of energy and water. Likewise, eating salt creates a dehydrated state that helps the animal retain additional water indirectly by increasing its fat stores. Both are ways an animal can stock up on crucial resources as a means to protect itself *before* it is in a desperate situation.

Nature is a genius. If only what is great for living in the wild were not such a bad thing in a society where sugar and salt are available on every dinner table.

Vasopressin: The Fat Hormone

Mild dehydration stimulates the development of obesity, and people with obesity show signs of dehydration. A high-salt diet is one way to trigger dehydration, and our studies showed that this, in turn, stimulates fructose production and fat formation. This suggests that the body's production of fructose represents a response to dehydration, similar to the release of vasopressin. Indeed, it appears that both function to protect us, with vasopressin acting to reduce water loss from the kidneys while fructose stimulates fat accumulation as a way to store water. In this way of thinking, vasopressin and fructose work in parallel to defend against dehydration. However, the two are much more connected in their effort to protect us from dehydration than we had imagined.

Fructose, as it turns out, directly stimulates the production of vasopressin. These two biologic responses, the production of fructose and the production of vasopressin, are not independent; rather, the production of vasopressin in response to dehydration is partially dependent on the production of fructose. In studies performed in our laboratory by physiologists Carlos Roncal and Zhilin Song, we found dehydration activates the polyol pathway in the brain, which generates fructose, which then stimulates vasopressin production. In fact, mice that lack the ability to metabolize fructose make less vasopressin when dehydrated. In other words, when we are dehydrated, the fructose we make not only helps us store water by making fat, but also helps us lose less water through our urine by increasing vasopressin production.

The fructose we eat or drink also stimulates vasopressin production. Our research team found that mice fed fructose develop high vasopressin levels even before they become obese, while this rise in vasopressin levels was not seen in mice that could not metabolize fructose.

Likewise, physiologist Zachary Schlader and colleagues showed that soft drinks raise blood vasopressin levels. And in a clinical study conducted by our collaborator Mehmet Kanbay from Koç University in Istanbul, we demonstrated that apple juice, which is rich in fructose, could also markedly increase vasopressin levels.

This made us wonder if the vasopressin itself might have a role in driving the survival switch. After all, vasopressin's job is to help us retain water, and stimulating fat production would be a good way to do that. It would also be consistent with why animals in the desert have both high vasopressin levels and excess fat, and why people who are overweight have high vasopressin levels. Many reports also suggest vasopressin could increase blood glucose and affect fat production; in particular, studies in obese rats by French physiologists Lise Bankir and Nadine Bouby had suggested vasopressin could play a role in insulin resistance and fatty liver.

To better understand vasopressin's involvement, Miguel and I designed a set of studies using mice that lacked **vasopressin receptors**. Hormones cause their effects by binding to receptors on cells. If vasopressin had a role in how fructose causes obesity, and we could block the ability of vasopressin to bind to its receptors, then the mice would not develop obesity and metabolic syndrome. Vasopressin is an especially complicated hormone, as it can bind to three different receptors, and the function of one of these, the V1b receptor, is not well understood. In studies led by endocrinologist Thomas Jensen and physiologist Ana Andres-Hernando in our laboratory, we found that mice that lacked the vasopressin V1b receptor (but still had the other receptors) were completely protected from developing obesity and metabolic syndrome. While we still do not fully understand the mechanism by which vasopressin causes obesity by binding to the V1b receptor, it is likely by stimulating other hormones and affecting fructose metabolism in the liver. In effect, vasopressin appears to amplify the switch.

Our discovery, in short, was that vasopressin is the fat hormone. It is responsible for how fructose drives obesity. And measuring it in the blood may be a useful way for predicting if we are at risk of developing obesity in the future.

One more interesting observation that emerged from our research, before we go on: drinking a beverage that contains fructose does not help fix dehydration, even though fructose encourages both water intake and formation of fat, which is an additional source of water. This is because fructose shifts water from the blood into cells (likely through increasing glycogen stores, as glycogen takes up water as it is made), leaving a high salt concentration behind and making you thirstier. Thus, soft drinks don't quench thirst, but rather leave us wanting more.

CAN DRINKING WATER TURN OFF THE SWITCH?

If obesity stems from a biological response to a dehydrated state and is driven by vasopressin, then could simple hydration with water provide a way to prevent or treat it?

There is a saying that, to be healthy, you should drink eight glasses of water a day, and many people carry water bottles with them all day long to stay hydrated. When I was in medical school, I considered this practice to be unnecessary. Our kidneys' job is to protect us from dehydration, I felt, and as long as we got a minimal amount of water (such as a few cups a day), if we started to get thirsty our kidneys would just release vasopressin to help us hold on to water. But that was before I knew that vasopressin not only reduces water loss through the kidneys, but also helps to increase our fat as a way to store water.

To study whether hydration could treat obesity, Masanari Kuwabara and Ana Andres-Hernando, who both were involved in our vasopressin studies, gave extra water to laboratory mice fed a high-sugar, high-fat diet. (This was done by hydrating their food, so that it was more like a gel than pellets.) The effect was dramatic. By doubling the animals' water intake, we could block obesity and insulin resistance. And even if we waited to increase the animals' water intake until after they were already fat, we could prevent further weight gain even if they continued on the high-sugar, high-fat diet.

A few studies in humans have studied whether increasing water intake also can help prevent obesity. The best have been performed in elementary schools and middle schools, where children were encouraged to drink more water through the installation of water fountains, and were shown frequent educational presentations on the importance of being well hydrated. Three different studies (one each in the United States, Germany, and England) showed that encouraging children to drink more water led to a reduction in obesity. In the study in Germany, the introduction of water fountains in schools led to an increase of just one glass of water per day, which in turn reduced children's risk of becoming overweight by 30 percent, compared to children in schools in which water fountains were not placed. A large study in Sweden, ongoing as of this writing, is seeking to determine if increased water intake can reduce obesity in adults, as well.

Staying well hydrated has always been recognized as important, but its importance in the prevention and treatment of obesity is just emerging.*

UMAMI: THE TASTE EVERYONE THOUGHT WAS SAFE

The discovery that sugar and salt activate the survival switch may not seem surprising in retrospect, for the simple reason that we are naturally attracted to sweet and salty foods. It makes sense that nature would have us seek them out,

---

* Before you change your drinking habits, be sure to read my recommendations in chapter nine. It is possible to drink too much water, which can be dangerous.

given that they either provide fructose directly or else stimulate its production (which both salt and dietary fructose do), thereby helping us store the critical fat we need for that rainy day when food cannot be found. Likewise, our bitter- and sour-sensing taste buds likely evolved to help us avoid foods more likely to be toxic.

In addition to our taste buds for salty, sweet, sour, and bitter flavors, we have a fifth type, **umami** (pronounced *oo-MA-mee*), which responds to foods with a savory flavor. Umami was originally identified in 1907 by Japanese chemist Kikunae Ikeda as the savory flavor present in sea kelp (kombu) and comes from the amino acid **glutamate**. Umami taste buds in our tongue sense glutamate present in foods and signal the brain to release dopamine much as sweetness does, creating a sense of pleasure.

Amino acids are the building blocks of protein, and glutamate can be released by ripening, aging, drying, curing, or cooking protein-containing foods. It is especially high in extracts from soy, fish, or yeast, and in tomatoes, especially dried tomatoes (it's why we like spaghetti sauce and Bloody Marys so much). The food industry has capitalized on our taste for umami by adding one form of glutamate, **monosodium glutamate** (**MSG**), to foods, especially pro- cessed meats and snack foods such as chips. Glutamate is generally considered safe, although high intake may cause headaches.

One cannot discuss umami without also mentioning that our taste for glu- tamate can be enhanced manifold by a set of substances identified by another Japanese researcher, who was studying why dried bonito* flakes enhance the taste of soups and other foods. These substances, AMP (adenosine monophos- phate) and IMP (**inosine monophosphate**), are present in high amounts in foods such as lobster and other shellfish, dark fish (mackerel, anchovies, and tuna), organ meats such as liver, and foods containing yeast (including several cheeses). Beer is especially high in umami, not because of the alcohol content, but because brewer's yeast is rich in glutamate as well as AMP and IMP.

Most studies have focused on umami foods—foods enriched in any of these three substances (glutamate, AMP, or IMP)†—as a way to enhance the flavor of

---

* A type of tuna.

† While some people view umami as only glutamate, our work suggests all three are taste enhancers that work alone or together, so I use the word umami to refer to any of these. Importantly, all three are commonly present in the same foods.

foods without the need to add sugar and salt. They are generally not thought of as having a role in causing obesity. However, some laboratory studies have found that glutamate can cause obesity in mice and cats. Even more concerning was a study of more than ten thousand Chinese adults that found a significant increased risk of obesity for those ingesting the most glutamate.

Miguel and I wondered whether these umami foods might also potentially engage the survival switch and provide an alternative way to increase fat stores and cause metabolic syndrome. Our reasoning was that, while glutamate has many functions in the body, including building and repairing proteins, it can also be used to make uric acid. Further, glutamate levels are also high in people with gout. And we have seen AMP before in this book: AMP is a key substance produced during the breakdown of our friend ATP, and plays an important part in how fructose drives the development of obesity and metabolic syndrome. Moreover, IMP is also involved in the survival switch, as AMP is broken down to IMP before uric acid is generated.

These observations raised the intriguing possibility that the reason we like the taste of glutamate, AMP, and IMP is that these substances are involved in the survival switch! This led us to reason that foods containing glutamate, AMP, and IMP might substitute for fructose and directly participate in the same chemical reaction that fructose uses to activate the survival switch. This means that they might be able to cause obesity and metabolic syndrome directly—no fructose required. In addition, we know uric acid can itself stimulate fructose production via the polyol pathway, and since all three of these substances can generate uric acid, umami foods also may be able to stimulate some fructose production as well.

Miguel and I tested this in our laboratory with a series of experiments in which laboratory mice were given MSG in their drinking water, with or without AMP or IMP. The results were exciting. Mice provided MSG (glutamate) lost control of their appetite and gained weight rapidly. They also had an increase in abdominal fat and developed insulin resistance. Similar results occurred in mice in a subsequent study that were given only AMP or only IMP. But the best way to get a mouse fat was to give both MSG with AMP or IMP.

Of course, this raised the question of whether the increased food intake and the development of obesity was in fact due to activation of the survival switch. Further studies suggested it was; we found that if we blocked the conversion of

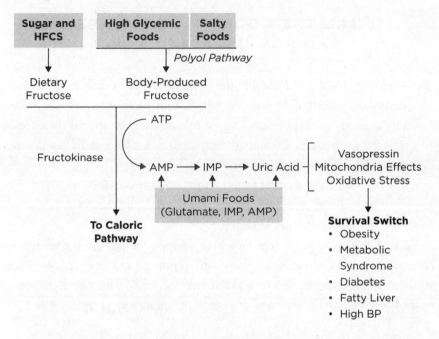

While sugar and HFCS are the dominant foods that turn on the survival switch, it can also be activated by high-glycemic carbohydrates, salty foods, and umami foods. All of these foods engage the energy depletion pathway, triggering the survival switch that results in obesity and metabolic syndrome.

glutamate to uric acid, we could also block weight gain. The same was true if we blocked the conversion of AMP and IMP to uric acid. The way umami causes obesity is by activating the survival switch—specifically, by directly engaging the **energy depletion pathway**.

Not only can glutamate cause obesity, but it was, in fact, stronger than either sugar or salt in doing so, gram for gram, in our studies with mice. However, we eat much less glutamate than we do sugar. The average American eats about 75 grams of fructose-containing sugars each day, but only half a gram of glutamate. Nevertheless, there are some individuals, especially in China, who are eating over 10 grams of glutamate a day in soy-based and other foods, and for them, the amount of umami consumed is likely contributing to weight gain.

Gram for gram, glutamate is more powerful than sugar or salt in causing obesity.

ALL THE FOODS WE LIKE ARE
BAD FOR US: WHAT NOW?

We now know that foods delivering the three flavors we most like—sweet, salt, and umami—all activate the survival switch. Our preference for these flavors probably evolved as a way to encourage us to seek, identify, and eat these foods; nature wants us to eat foods that will help us store fat. One could say that our biology makes doing so a natural instinct.

Jack LaLanne,* the original fitness guru, famously commented, "If it tastes good, spit it out." I do not know your opinion, but I find the evidence that the foods we like make us fat discouraging.

But there's some good news. We have options; we can use the science we have learned to develop effective plans both to prevent and treat obesity. Before we dive in there, however, let's first take a closer look at how the switch influences other diseases besides obesity and diabetes—including some surprising ones.

---

* Jack claimed that in his younger life he was a "sugar-aholic"—that he was addicted to sugar like some people are to alcohol. We will learn more about the interesting relationship of sugar and alcohol in chapter seven.

PART II

The Fat Switch and Disease

CHAPTER 6

The Bread-and-Butter Diseases of Humankind

O ver the last century or so—ever since that 1893 World's Fair—sugar intake, already high, has continued to rise worldwide. Not surprisingly, there has also been a dramatic rise in obesity and metabolic syndrome, as well as diabetes, hypertension, stroke, and heart disease. In addition, there has been a rise in cancers associated with obesity, including breast, colon, and pancreatic cancers.

The parallel rise in all of these diseases is well appreciated in popular and medical literature, and the conditions are closely interrelated. Certainly there are common risk factors, many associated with Western culture and diet. However, it is complicated and difficult to discern which of the many causes that have been suggested is, or are, responsible. Is it as simple as lack of exercise, or eating too much, or a specific food? How important is socioeconomic status, or our genetics, or exposure to toxins, or what happened to our mothers while we were in the womb? Perhaps with the proper weighting we could develop an equation that took all these factors into account to accurately sum up an individual's risk for developing disease. Or could it be much simpler than that? Could there be one major underlying mechanism driving the whole shebang?

In the fourteenth century, a Franciscan friar and theologian, William of Ockham, proposed that, in problem-solving, the simplest explanation is often the right one. His teachings became known as Ockham's razor, a philosophical tenet commonly used in medicine. Could Ockham's razor be applied to find an underlying cause driving not just obesity, metabolic syndrome, and diabetes, but also hypertension, stroke, heart disease, liver and kidney diseases, and more? Specifically, could persistent activation of our recently discovered survival switch be the root cause not only of obesity and diabetes, but also of these associated noncommunicable diseases? Is there evidence to support this hypothesis, and, if proven, would it change how we view these conditions and what we do to prevent or manage these diseases?

There is, of course, danger in oversimplifying a problem. To argue that the switch may be the cause of many of the more important diseases of the day might sound presumptuous and even fanatical. Yet there is an attractiveness to simplicity in biology as well as other fields, and so it is reasonable to explore this idea more deeply. Perhaps what matters most is to determine not if the switch is the *primary* cause, but rather if it is a *contributory* cause. The latter idea may be easier to accept and is still important, for, so long as the switch has a role, then developing strategies to block its activation might provide new insights into disease prevention, disease management, and potential cures.

Let's begin by looking at many of the diseases associated with obesity and metabolic syndrome, and seeing whether they could be related to the survival switch.

GOUT: THE POSTER CHILD FOR ACTIVATION OF THE SURVIVAL SWITCH

There is probably no disease that better exemplifies the persistent activation of the survival switch than gout. As you may recall from chapter three, gout is a type of arthritis* in which people become seized with pain, typically in the big toe, ankle, or knee. The joint becomes hot and red, and the pain can be so severe that even a bedsheet over the foot causes discomfort. It is one of the

---

* Latin for "inflammation in the joints."

most common types of arthritis worldwide, and affects 9 million people in the United States.

Gout is caused by elevated blood levels of uric acid, typically higher than 7 mg/dL. Uric acid is not very soluble, and if blood levels get too high, crystals can form and be deposited in the joints, which elicits inflammation (causing the painful arthritis). Less commonly, uric acid crystals also form under the skin, where they tend to form small, painless nodules called tophi. The classic gout attack occurs late at night or early in the morning after a rich meal, one that typically includes alcohol, red meat (rich in glutamate and the **nucleotides** AMP and IMP), and sugar. And it is especially common in people with sleep apnea, because the fall in blood oxygen levels they experience during sleep further increases the production of uric acid in the body.

Most gout attacks last five to ten days and resolve with anti-inflammatory drugs, but the disease often recurs, and may lead to joint deformities. Because it responds so well to over-the-counter medications, physicians and patients often view gout as more of a nuisance than as a disease, with the result that it has not received the attention it deserves.

However, gout is much more than just a bothersome arthritis you take ibuprofen for when a twinge of pain suggests an attack is imminent. Rather, it is, in most cases, the poster child for persistent activation of the survival switch.

You might recall from chapter four that humans have higher uric acid levels than most other mammals because of a mutation in the gene for uricase that occurred millions of years ago. Initially, that mutation only led to a modest rise in the normal range of uric acid, from 1–2 mg/dL to about 3–4 mg/dL. However, the introduction of the Western diet, and especially alcohol and foods rich in sugar and umami, has pushed uric acid even higher, so that average levels today are 5–6 mg/dL—and the uric acid of as many as 20 million people in the US is even higher. These elevated levels (>6 mg/dL in women and >7 mg/dL in men) are sometimes referred to as **hyperuricemia**, and people with hyperuricemia are the ones most likely to develop gout.

While high uric acid levels can have several causes, including genetics and kidney failure, high levels and/or the presence of gout strongly suggest a diet rich in foods that activate the survival switch, because uric acid is one of the main products of fructose metabolism. It should therefore not be a surprise that subjects with gout have some of the highest rates of obesity and metabolic syndrome in the world. Nearly three-quarters of patients with gout have high blood pressure, more than half are obese, more than half have chronic kidney disease, the majority have fatty liver, and one-quarter have type 2 diabetes. People with gout also have some of the highest rates of heart disease.

This suggests that the presence of gout, or of elevated uric acid (i.e., hyperuricemia), is another consequence of the survival switch in overdrive. However, our experimental data suggested an interesting twist: that uric acid is not simply a by-product of the survival switch, but also an active participant in triggering it. Beyond causing oxidative stress to the energy factories, it may have other biological effects, including stimulating fat production, inflammation, and blood vessel constriction. There is strong evidence in laboratory animals that uric acid has a role in driving high blood pressure, insulin resistance, fatty liver, and obesity. Indeed, recall that the reason we originally became interested in fructose was a study that found lowering uric acid levels could improve the metabolic syndrome in rats that were fed fructose. These observations suggest that uric acid may have a role in driving weight gain, elevated blood pressure, insulin resistance, and other features of metabolic syndrome.

This viewpoint—that uric acid is a contributor to metabolic disease—is currently controversial, as for years we believed that uric acid rises in response to obesity, insulin resistance, and high blood pressure, or from treatments of these conditions (especially diuretics used to control blood pressure). However, there are a number of arguments that favor uric acid as having a contributory role in these diseases. First, there is good evidence that high uric acid precedes the development of obesity, metabolic syndrome, and these related conditions, and if it precedes these conditions, then we cannot state that its presence is solely a consequence of them. For example, in one study we followed healthy Japanese adults whose only abnormality was high uric acid levels, along with a control group with normal uric acid levels. After five years, the subjects with high uric acid had double the risk of developing high blood pressure, diabetes, obesity, and chronic kidney disease. There are dozens of studies of the general population as well that show high uric acid can independently predict the development of these conditions, as well as heart disease.

There is also evidence that lowering uric acid can prevent or reverse features of metabolic syndrome. Some of the strongest evidence relates to blood pressure. In a study performed with our collaborator Daniel Feig, a pediatric nephrologist, we looked at the effects of lowering uric acid on adolescent patients with newly diagnosed high blood pressure. Our research group had previously shown in laboratory animals that high blood pressure is most responsive to lowering uric acid early on. Over time, high uric acid causes progressive injury to and inflammation in the kidneys, such that the high blood pressure is eventually driven by the kidneys rather than uric acid directly; when this happens, lowering uric acid becomes less effective. Therefore, we thought this group of patients would be an ideal test group, as they would have minimal kidney disease at the time. To our amazement, when Dan measured the patients' uric acid, the vast majority (90 percent) had high levels. Dan then did a randomized study and found that using allopurinol (one of the more potent uric acid–lowering drugs) for uric acid reduction could completely reverse hypertension, whereas the placebo had no effect. When he performed a similar study in overweight adolescents with borderline hypertension, he again found that lowering uric acid could restore blood pressure to normal, while the placebo had no effect.

We found similar benefits of lowering uric acid on blood pressure while working with other collaborators, including Mexican nephrologist and clinical researcher Magdalena Madero, and Turkish nephrologist Mehmet Kanbay. Mehmet also showed that lowering uric acid could improve insulin resistance in subjects with high uric acid levels, as did other researchers. Further, lowering uric acid seemed to have beneficial effects on weight, and especially on preventing weight gain. In one of Dan's studies, for example, adolescents on a placebo gained five pounds during the course of the study, while the group receiving allopurinol actually lost one pound.

While these and many other studies have shown that lowering uric acid levels has beneficial effects on metabolic syndrome, some studies have not. However, these negative results can usually be ascribed to one of two things. First, a number of these studies lowered uric acid in subjects whose uric acid levels were already normal. Others wanted to know if lowering uric acid might treat high blood pressure but performed the study in subjects with normal blood pressure. These types of studies do not make much sense to me, as it is testing a treatment in people who do not need treating.

In addition to having a potential role in metabolic syndrome, uric acid may have a direct role in heart disease, especially in patients with gout. Recent studies suggest that uric acid crystals do not just deposit in the joints of patients with gout, but also may do silent harm in other parts of the body, too. One study, for example, found that nearly 80 percent of people with gout have uric acid crystals in their heart and blood vessels; they are also commonly present in the kidneys. Since the crystals can cause local inflammation, it raises the strong possibility that this is one way overactivation of the switch causes heart and kidney disease (see the following sections for more). Clearly, we need more clinical trials to understand the full implications of high uric acid levels and gout.*

Gout is a systemic disease that exemplifies the negative health impacts of sending the survival switch into overdrive.

Gout is not simply an annoyance. It is a systemic disease that exemplifies the negative health impacts of sending the survival switch into overdrive. But what about the individual diseases such as diabetes that are so common today? Could the fat switch be a contributory cause of these disorders, too?

TYPE 2 DIABETES: ENDGAME OF INSULIN RESISTANCE

Diabetes is a condition in which blood sugar (glucose) levels are abnormally elevated. There are two kinds: **type 1**, which occurs when the pancreas loses the ability to make insulin and usually develops during childhood; and **type 2**, which is associated with obesity and metabolic syndrome. Type 2 diabetes is by far more common, and the type associated with one of the chief characteristics of the survival switch: insulin resistance.

Subjects who develop type 2 diabetes typically show evidence of insulin resistance prior to developing full-blown diabetes. In this setting, the muscle is resistant to the effects of insulin, and the pancreas produces more insulin to compensate, increasing levels until there is enough to overcome the resistance.

---

* There are now many trials evaluating the potential benefit of lowering uric acid on heart disease. Some are ongoing. Others are detailed further in chapter nine.

This reduces the blood glucose, but as a consequence, circulating insulin levels remain high. The pancreas also has to work overtime, and over time, low-grade inflammation in the pancreas can cause scarring, compromising the pancreas's ability to produce insulin. As insulin levels fall, blood glucose can no longer be controlled, and diabetes develops.

While the exact mechanism for the development of insulin resistance is still being determined, it is clear from our and others' research that insulin resistance is linked to the metabolism of fructose, that it represents a consequence of survival switch activation, and that the mechanism likely involves effects of uric acid. Our group also found that the administration of sucrose to rats led to frank diabetes, in which the insulin-producing cells in the pancreas were damaged. In other words, type 2 diabetes appears to develop as a direct consequence of the metabolism of fructose, which causes both the insulin resistance and the damage to the pancreas that culminate in the diabetic state. This does not mean that there are not other causes of type 2 diabetes, but that fructose appears to be the primary one.

The evidence that fructose-containing sugars are a cause of type 2 diabetes is overwhelming. The earliest comes from history. You may recall from chapter four that one of the first reports of diabetes in the literature was by Sushruta, a physician who practiced in the Ganges River Valley during history's earliest sugarcane harvests, and who linked obesity and diabetes with the liquid cane sugar they drank. In the rest of the world, diabetes remained relatively rare until sugar intake increased in the late Renaissance. In the 1800s, the French physician Étienne Lancereaux realized that there were two types of diabetes, "lean" and "obese," and recognized that the latter was commonly associated with sugar intake. By the early 1900s, a rise in diabetes was being observed throughout the world and increasingly being linked with sugar intake.

One of the strongest associations of sugar intake with diabetes was found by Haven Emerson, New York City health commissioner between 1915 and 1918. Emerson became concerned about the steady increase in diabetes in the city; in a span of forty years it had risen about tenfold, from two to three cases per one hundred thousand in 1880 to nearly twenty cases per one hundred thousand in 1920. To investigate the reason, he performed a large survey of the populace, looking for potential risk factors. He found that diabetes was most associated with being overweight and sedentary, but he also noted a remarkable association with sugar intake. At that time sugar was still expensive, and diabetes was almost exclusively a rich man's disease.

Emerson was not alone. Others at the time also believed sugar to be the cause of diabetes, especially Frederick Banting, the physician who shared the Nobel Prize for discovering insulin. However, not everyone was in agreement. One of the more vocal opponents was the physician Elliott Joslin. An expert on diabetes, Joslin rejected the idea that sugar was the cause and proposed it was overnutrition instead. He noted that a study that evaluated the relationship between sugar consumption from 1923 and 1928 and the mortality rate from diabetes did not find a strong correlation. However, of the thirteen countries in the study with the highest sugar consumption, eleven also appeared in the top thirteen for diabetic mortality rates. And while the other two (then) countries, Cuba and Hawaii, had relatively low diabetic mortality rates, there is often a ten- to twenty-year delay between a rise in sugar intake and an increase in diabetic mortality, and during the decade following the study, diabetes rates and diabetes mortality rates in Hawaii soared. (Regarding Cuba, it is unclear how reliable the original data collection was.)

Today, the association of diabetes with sugar and HFCS intake—especially from soft drinks—is strongly supported by both laboratory and clinical studies. Consuming fructose can induce diabetes in laboratory animals and insulin resistance in humans. Reducing fructose intake also has been reported to lessen insulin resistance in people with obesity. Today there is no doubt that fructose, and therefore the survival switch, plays an important role in causing this disease.

Reducing fructose intake also lessens insulin resistance in people with obesity.

Sugar is not the only food associated with diabetes risk, but as we've seen, sugar is not the only food that turns on the survival switch, even if it is its major driver. It is therefore not surprising that high-glycemic carbohydrates, including foods such as rice and potatoes, also increase the risk for diabetes, although not as strongly. The same is true for red meat, beer, and other umami foods, and for high-salt diets. All of these data suggest that type 2 diabetes is an unwanted gift of the fat switch.

HYPERTENSION, HEART FAILURE, AND STROKE

High blood pressure, or hypertension, is usually defined as a blood pressure of 140/90 mm Hg or higher, although in recent years there has been some move to change the threshold to 130/80 mm Hg. Similar to obesity and diabetes, it used to be a rare condition, and in the 1890s was thought to afflict less than 5 percent of the US adult population. But just like obesity and diabetes, it increased in the twentieth century; today, one-third of adults in the US suffer from the condition. It is now one of the most common diseases worldwide, affecting more than 1 billion adults.

Hypertension is called "the silent killer" because it usually has few, if any, symptoms. Many people are unaware that they have it, and so go untreated; others go inadequately treated. Yet high blood pressure takes a brutal toll on the body. First, it causes the heart to work harder than it should, which in the long term can lead to heart failure; today, high blood pressure is its number-one cause. High blood pressure also gradually damages blood vessels. One place this damage can occur is the brain. Hypertension can cause blood vessels to break, leading to intracranial bleeding. It can also cause blood vessels to narrow, reducing blood supply to parts of the brain and causing them to die. Big blood vessels, such as the aorta, are vulnerable as well. High blood pressure there can cause aneurysms that can result in internal bleeding or dissection, the latter a horrific complication in which the lining of the big vessels suddenly rips. Furthermore, high blood pressure is one of the major causes of kidney failure, and can result in other problems. For example, it can adversely affect school performance in kids and cause slowly progressive dementia, called vascular dementia, in older people via damage to the small vessels in the brain.

There is an urgent need to understand all causes of high blood pressure. While some causes are well known, such as kidney disease, the vast majority of cases are labeled as "primary hypertension" or "essential hypertension," meaning the cause is not known. However, there is increasing evidence that primary hypertension is due to overactivation of the survival switch.

There is strong evidence that fructose may play a role in hypertension. Epidemiological studies have linked intake of soft drinks, as well as intake of fructose from added sugars, with high blood pressure. Even stronger evidence is the finding that volunteers develop an immediate rise in blood pressure after they are given fructose, whereas this is not observed with glucose or water. In one clinical trial we were involved in, participants were randomly assigned to drink a soft drink containing either sucrose or HFCS, where the only difference in the drinks was the added sugar each contained. Both drinks caused a rise in blood pressure, but the HFCS caused a greater rise, correlating both with HFCS's slightly higher fructose content and a greater rise in uric acid level.

That correlation with uric acid level turns out to be important, something we verified in a study performed with clinician Enrique Perez-Pozo. Male volunteers, half of whom were randomly selected to receive allopurinol, drank large amounts of fructose daily for two weeks. Blood pressure increased markedly in the group given fructose, but this rise in blood pressure in response to fructose intake was *completely blocked* in the allopurinol group, in whom a rise in uric acid was prevented. These data suggest that activation of the survival switch by fructose plays a role in blood pressure, and that it likely involves the effect of fructose in raising uric acid levels.

The substance to which hypertension has traditionally been linked is not sugar, of course, but salt. The survival switch can also be activated by a high-salt diet, but as we've discussed, this is due not to the salt itself, but rather to a rise in salt concentration in the blood, which triggers production of fructose and the hormone vasopressin. To test this effect on blood pressure, our collaborator, Mehmet Kanbay, gave volunteers a salty soup to drink, either with or without two glasses of drinking water. If the subjects drank only the soup, the concentration of salt in their blood and their blood pressure, along with vasopressin, rose immediately. However, if the subjects ingested the water as they did salty soup, no increase in salt concentration was observed and no change in vasopressin or blood pressure occurred.

This and other similar studies suggest it is not the amount of salt we eat that raises blood pressure, but rather whether the salt we eat causes a rise in the salt concentration in our blood that activates the survival switch. We confirmed this in a study with our collaborator Masanari Kuwabara, a Japanese cardiologist, where we evaluated the relationship of salt intake to the development of high blood pressure in a large, healthy Japanese population. We found that while higher daily salt intake does predict an increased risk of high blood pressure after five years, the stronger predictor was not the amount of salt ingested, but rather the concentration of salt in the blood.

Just as the intake of added sugars has increased in the last decades, so has the intake of salt—by 30 percent. Salt restriction has become a standard recommendation for lowering blood pressure, and is now being recognized as a strategy to reduce weight, too. Yet our research shows that it is not really the amount of salt that is important in driving blood pressure, but the balance of salt and water. Accordingly, if we can keep fructose intake low, and drink plenty of water to help prevent our blood salt concentration from getting high, we have a good chance of preventing hypertension without restricting salt too severely.

While the survival switch's release of uric acid and vasopressin is what increases blood pressure in the short term, there is evidence that another system eventually takes over. Specifically, activating the survival switch results in low-grade inflammation in the kidneys, and work led by my collaborator Bernardo Rodriguez-Iturbe, a leader in the field of hypertension, has shown that over time this inflammation becomes self-perpetuating. The inflammation causes the kidneys to retain salt, which results in persistently elevated blood pressure. This is likely the case for individuals who have been hypertensive for many years. When this happens, just lowering uric acid or turning off the switch will not cure high blood pressure. Nevertheless, reducing intake of added sugars and salt should still provide some benefit, as turning off the survival switch will help prevent things from getting worse.

It is not the amount of salt that is important in driving blood pressure, but the balance of salt and water.

LIVER DISEASE

In the 1970s, doctors began to see a new type of liver disease that has since increased dramatically throughout the world. Today it is the most common cause of liver failure and the need for a liver transplant. The disease is called non-alcoholic fatty liver disease, sometimes referred to as NAFLD. It is also a silent killer. The first stage is an accumulation of fat in the liver, leading to some mild enlargement and, commonly, mildly abnormal liver function tests. At this stage the individual is usually unaware that there is anything wrong unless the physician notes the presence of fatty liver from some type of imaging, such as ultrasound. Over time, localized low-grade inflammation develops—which, again, carries no symptoms. Unnoticed, the inflammation causes damage and scarring. Then, typically years later, the individual suddenly presents with signs of liver failure, called cirrhosis. The patient may be confused, with tremors, muscle loss, a great swelling in the abdomen from fluid, and sometimes bleeding in the gut. Once this happens, there is very little that can be done except a liver transplant.

The disease appears very similar to alcohol-related liver disease, as alcohol also causes fatty liver that over time is associated with inflammation, scarring, and cirrhosis. In fact, the two conditions are almost identical, although the latter often is a bit more dramatic in presentation and, of course, is associated with heavy alcohol use.

It is very likely that NAFLD is a direct consequence of continual activation of the survival switch. As you may recall, one of the main functions of the survival switch is to accumulate fat, and while adipose tissues are one favored place, the liver is another.

Fatty liver can be a good thing, as it can be a storage site for fuel. Recall the hummingbird, which lives off nectar and develops the fattiest liver of all birds, only to burn off that fat during the night. Fructose's ability to cause fatty liver in birds has been known since the time of Rome. Pliny the Elder wrote that the Roman chef Marcus Apicus would feed geese dates to give them fatty liver, which over time became a famous delicacy, foie gras, that we continue to eat today. Modern laboratory studies have shown that feeding fructose to other animals causes fatty liver in them, as well.

Back in 2006, when I was still at the University of Florida, I had the opportunity to attend a lecture on NAFLD given by Manal Abdelmalek, a brilliant young physician who was studying this relatively new disease. As she presented, it struck me that NAFLD might be developing from the consumption of foods or drinks containing HFCS and sucrose. After the lecture, we talked; she told me that no one had specifically considered this possibility, and so we began a collaboration. On interviewing her subjects with NAFLD, she found that they had a remarkable history of drinking excessive amounts of soft drinks containing

HFCS, and most of them had features of metabolic syndrome and high uric acid levels. Xiaosen Ouyang from our laboratory also examined liver biopsies from these individuals and found that the expression of enzymes involved in the metabolism of fructose (particularly fructokinase) was very high. It seemed like we had a strong case that NAFLD resulted from intake of added sugars containing fructose.

Subsequently, Manal showed in a series of beautifully designed studies that intake of soft drinks containing HFCS predicted not only the development of fatty liver, but also the inflammation and scarring that could lead to cirrhosis. She further showed that fatty liver cells were chronically depleted of energy (ATP)—a telltale sign of the survival switch at work—and that ATP levels were inversely correlated with fructose intake and uric acid levels. Since then, numerous studies have linked NAFLD with excessive intake of added sugars. One study even reported that reducing intake of added sugars improved fatty liver in children.

With the association between added sugars and fatty liver proven, we began wondering whether there was any difference in the ability of HFCS to cause fatty liver compared to sucrose, as the appearance of NAFLD correlated most with the introduction of HFCS. We looked at this by giving laboratory rats either sucrose or an HFCS mixture with a 50:50 fructose-to-glucose ratio, so that each group received the same amount of fructose. Our study found that the HFCS mixture caused more severe fatty liver than the sucrose, although sucrose also increased fat and caused liver inflammation. A third, control group on a normal diet did not develop fatty liver at all.

Anyone who has fatty liver, or a diagnosis of NAFLD, should beware that the primary cause of their condition is very likely from added sugars containing fructose. HFCS appears to be more potent than sucrose, possibly because of differences in absorption, as sucrose must first be separated into fructose and glucose prior to absorption by the gut. However, this does not exonerate sucrose, which should still be viewed as a major risk factor.

CHRONIC KIDNEY DISEASE

As with the other diseases we've considered in this chapter, chronic kidney disease has increased over the last century in parallel with obesity. One reason is that the incidence of chronic kidney disease is especially high in people with metabolic syndrome, and the two most common causes of kidney failure are diabetes and high blood pressure. Since both diabetes and hypertension appear to result from activation of the survival switch, it is likely that kidney disease is another indirect casualty.

However, there is evidence that fructose may *directly* cause kidney damage, too. The kidney, along with the liver and brain, metabolizes fructose, and the resultant uric acid causes local inflammation and oxidative stress. We have found that high-fructose diets can cause kidney damage over time and can also accelerate preexisting kidney damage. We also have found that the kidney can make fructose via the polyol pathway, especially in the setting of diabetes, and that this can lead to kidney damage, too—likely part of why diabetes causes kidney disease.

Finally, the survival switch is known to raise uric acid levels, and numerous studies have reported that such elevated levels predict the development of chronic kidney disease. Other studies have reported that lowering uric acid can slow the progression of chronic kidney disease in subjects with elevated levels or with gout. Recently, these findings were called in question by two highly publicized studies that did not show a benefit, but neither study included subjects with gout (the individuals most likely to benefit), and both studies included subjects with normal uric acid levels (who would not be expected to benefit) in addition to subjects with high uric acid levels. Further studies to address this question are needed.

ATHEROSCLEROSIS, HEART ATTACKS, AND SUDDEN DEATH

Most people who develop heart disease—distinct from heart failure due to long-standing high blood pressure, discussed earlier—do so as a result of coronary artery disease. This condition is usually caused by atherosclerosis, the buildup of cholesterol-rich fat deposits in the arteries that supply blood to the heart and other organs. These plaques are sites where clots can form and obstruct blood flow and oxygen delivery. The clots and plaque debris may also become dislodged and end up in the brain or elsewhere, causing heart attack or stroke.

For years we've known that family history, high cholesterol levels, and smoking are major risk factors for atherosclerosis. Recently, researchers have also recognized persistent low-grade inflammation as an additional risk factor—something heavily associated with the survival switch.

While severe inflammation is never a good thing, chronic low-grade inflammation can help our body defend against some infections, as it tends to make it easier for our white blood cells to kill bacteria and parasites. One major cause of low-grade inflammation is uric acid, making inflammation another likely benefit of the survival switch. However, when the switch is in overdrive, this low-grade inflammation ceases to be beneficial. For example, low-grade inflammation in our blood vessels is responsible for the development of cholesterol-rich atherosclerotic plaques. Uric acid and its crystals have been identified in these plaques in many patients with gout, so it seems likely they are playing a role in the damage occurring there.

The full role of fructose and uric acid in coronary artery disease is still unknown. More clinical studies are needed, but it seems likely that heart disease might be another downstream complication of the fat switch.

CANCER

As noted at the start of this chapter, obesity is associated with several cancers, including cancer of the breast, colon, and pancreas. Why obesity should be associated with cancer has been a mystery. However, the answer may not be that obesity causes cancer, but rather that chronic activation of the survival switch increases the risk for both obesity and cancer.

You may remember from chapter three that the survival switch not only stimulates fat accumulation to store energy and water, but also protects animals in situations where oxygen levels are low. When oxygen levels fall, the body starts making fructose via the polyol pathway. This fructose then causes oxidative stress, as part of the survival switch, which dampens the function of the mitochondria. Since the mitochondria use oxygen to make energy, a reduction in energy production by the mitochondria also leads to a reduction in our oxygen needs. The decrease in energy production by the mitochondria is compensated for by the stimulation of **glycolysis**, a more primitive and less efficient method of making energy, which does not require oxygen.

This is how the naked mole rat of Africa survives in its crowded burrows deep underground, where oxygen levels can get very low. It produces large amounts of fructose to minimize its oxygen needs, such that it can live for up to five hours in air that contains only 5 percent oxygen,* where a mouse could survive only about ten minutes. I suspect other animals also survive low oxygen conditions by making fructose via the polyol pathway—animals such as the elephant seal, which can hold its breath and dive for up to forty minutes, and birds that can fly at exceptional heights, such as the bar-headed goose, which has flown over the Himalayas.

As with the other benefits of the survival switch, the ability to use fructose to help survive low-oxygen conditions has an ironic twist: today, it may be a detriment to our survival by increasing our cancer risk. Many cancer cells have to survive under low-oxygen conditions. For example, when a cancer first spreads to new tissue, it has to survive under low oxygen conditions until it can form the little blood vessels needed to provide oxygen and nutrients to help it grow. Fructose is cancer cells' preferred fuel, for it supports tumor growth under these low-oxygen conditions. HFCS, for example, has been shown to accelerate the growth of intestinal tumors in mice due to the effects of fructose on reducing oxygen needs. Some cancer cells, such as metastatic colon cancer, pancreatic cancer, and breast cancer, particularly like fructose as a fuel, and this may explain why these cancers are more common in individuals with obesity.

There is now active interest in determining whether low-fructose diets can slow or prevent cancer spread. Researchers are also evaluating whether products of fructose metabolism, such as uric acid and lactic acid, may have a role in stimulating tumor growth and spread. For example, a study led by one of my collaborators, biologist Mehdi Fini, found that mice lacking uricase, if injected with breast cancer cells, experience much more rapid tumor growth and spread compared to normal mice.

Thus, it seems that, while the survival switch might not cause cancer, fructose and the switch may encourage cancer cells' survival and growth.

---

* For contrast, the available oxygen content of air at sea level is about 21 percent, and at the top of Everest is about 7 percent.

It is striking how many modern diseases may have resulted at least partly from excessive intake of fructose-containing sugars or foods that result in the production of fructose in the body. Nature must be dismayed. What aided survival in one setting has become maladaptive in another, wreaking havoc on our health. Unfortunately, there is another entire area of medicine that the survival switch can influence—and that is not diseases of the body, but of the brain.

CHAPTER 7

How the Survival Switch Affects Our Mind and Behavior

O ver-engagement of the survival switch appears instrumental in many of today's most widespread diseases. Yet fructose may have far-reaching effects on another aspect of our health, one with equally severe consequences, and that is our mind and our behavior. Recall that one of the major actions of the survival switch involves stimulating hunger, craving, and foraging for food. When these behaviors are put into overdrive, our survival responses can become behavioral disorders. And while some of the evidence is currently limited to associations or initial reports, together it suggests that fructose can affect our behavior; our mental faculties, including our risk for dementia; and even our desire for a glass of wine.

ADDICTION AND ALCOHOLISM

Many people find sugar addicting. I am one of them. I crave sugar even though I know it is bad for me. I can dream all day long of chocolate fudge cake with whipped cream, strawberry shortcake, and homemade apple pie with vanilla ice cream. I am, in the words of the late fitness guru Jack LaLanne, a sugar-aholic. It does not matter that I have spent my life doing research that has identified sugar as a major cause of diabetes and other diseases. I still love sugar.

I am not alone in my love affair with sugar. My children love it as well. The craving for sugar is innate, governed by the sweet taste buds on our tongue that signal pleasure to the brain every time we taste it. Babies prefer sugar over breast milk.* Sugar is part of the vocabulary of love, from "sweetheart" to "honey bear." Sugar is what makes the medicine go down, and most people look forward to birthday cake. And what could be better than having a "Golden Ticket" to Willy Wonka's chocolate factory? Whether it is beautiful ballet (the "Dance of the Sugar Plum Fairy") or rock 'n' roll ("Brown Sugar" by the Rolling Stones), sugar is always finding a way into our life.

The craving for sucrose and high-fructose corn syrup is not simply a preference for sweetness, for as we explained earlier, animals that lack the ability to taste them still prefer sucrose and HFCS over foods without these added sugars. Sucrose is special in its ability to entice us to eat it.

Our love for sugars such as sucrose and HFCS can turn into a true addiction. This is best shown in animals when sugars are given intermittently, such as by providing laboratory rats sugary water only at night. The animals will wait in anticipation for their sugar water, and even fight over who gets to it first. Over time they drink more each day, much as we see in animals addicted to drugs. This is not that surprising, because studies have found that sucrose and HFCS stimulate the same parts of the brain as heroin. If the evening sugary water is no longer provided, the rats become agitated, huddle in a corner with their hair on end, or show other signs of withdrawal. Evidence that this represents a true withdrawal syndrome was shown by Bart Hoebel, a physiologist known for his studies on sugar craving. He found that laboratory rats fed sugar also undergo withdrawal following the injection of naloxone, a drug that blocks

Sucrose and HFCS stimulate the same parts of the brain as heroin.

* Breast milk does contain a kind of sugar, lactose, but it does not contain fructose.

the effects of opiates in the brain and can precipitate withdrawal in patients addicted to heroin.

While sugar acts similarly to heroin in its ability to cause addiction, there is an especially close relationship between sugar and another drug: alcohol. Robert Lustig, a physician who is an expert on sugar and fructose, has written that sugar is like "alcohol without the buzz," because both sugar and alcohol provide pleasure, and both can be addicting. He has additionally noted that both fructose and alcohol also cause fatty liver disease and cirrhosis. Indeed, as we saw last chapter, multiple studies have shown that liver disease caused by one substance is almost indistinguishable from that caused by the other.

It should not be that surprising, then, to learn that heavy drinkers show a stronger than normal craving for sweet drinks compared to subjects who do not drink much alcohol. Likewise, a history of alcoholism in the parents, especially the father, is associated with a stronger than usual craving for sugar in children.

This suggests that, when an alcoholic stops drinking, such as when they are admitted to the hospital with an alcohol-associated complication, they might seek to appease their craving for alcohol by drinking soft drinks or eating a lot of sugary foods. Indeed, when I round at the hospital, I find that patients admitted with alcohol-associated liver failure almost inevitably have multiple soft drinks on the bed table adjacent to their bed. (This is especially bad since, if you have liver failure, the last thing you should do is drink soft drinks, as they will only make the liver disease worse.)

Cravings for sugar and alcohol are definitely intertwined. Experimental studies show that animals addicted to sucrose will also drink more alcohol if it is offered. Indeed, a simple way to increase alcohol intake is to add sucrose to it, which also results in a much more rapid development of liver disease. This is worrisome as many people add sucrose to make mixed drinks such as margaritas or piña coladas, while some other alcohols are naturally sweet from residual sugars, such as rum, port, and Madeira wine. The presence of sugar in these drinks not only makes them additionally appealing, but also likely stimulates more alcohol intake, translating into a greater risk for sugar and alcohol complications.

The fact that sugar and alcohol are commonly interchanged or combined turns out to be more than just a coincidence. If we put on our detective hats once more, there is an important clue, one that has to do with alcohol's ability to cause dehydration.

You've probably heard that, when you've been drinking, you should be sure to drink a lot of water before you go to bed, because it helps reduce the risk of a morning headache from dehydration. Alcohol causes dehydration not only because it makes us urinate more but also because when it accumulates in the blood, the sum concentrations of the salt and alcohol become high relative to the water present. This is similar to what happens in response to a high-salt diet, and the body reacts by sensing this as dehydration and triggering thirst. Since dehydration stimulates the body to make fructose, this suggests that drinking alcohol might be another way to make fructose. Could this be one reason alcohol is so attractive?

To test alcohol's potential role in fructose production, Miguel Lanaspa from our group gave alcohol to laboratory mice. As the mice drank more and more alcohol, they became dehydrated. As we'd suspected, this activated the polyol pathway, resulting in high concentrations of fructose in the liver, even though the mice were not eating any fructose. Alcohol stimulates fructose production.

As you may recall from the last chapter, fructose causes *non*-alcoholic fatty liver disease (or NAFLD), while alcohol causes alcohol-associated fatty liver disease. However, as also mentioned earlier, the two are almost identical in appearance. This led us to wonder whether alcohol causes liver disease *because* it stimulates fructose production. To test this, we gave alcohol to mice that could not break down fructose. Amazingly, the alcohol failed to cause liver disease. In other words, fructose is also the cause of alcohol-induced liver disease.

We were in for yet another surprise, however. Specifically, we found that intake of alcohol was dramatically less in the mice that could not metabolize fructose. They drank less than one-quarter of the alcohol a normal mouse does. This suggests that the craving for alcohol is related to the craving for fructose.

This finding is significant because of its implications for treating alcoholism—a serious worldwide problem that can affect many aspects of a person's life, including work, friends, family, and of course health. Most often, people combat alcoholism through counseling, joining community groups like Alcoholics Anonymous, or entering drug treatment programs. Some medications have been developed, but most of them work on various substances in the brain that drive craving, and they can have undesirable side effects. But if we find a way to block fructose metabolism, we may be able to cure alcoholism.* Just restricting sugar intake may also help reduce the craving for alcohol, though this has not yet been evaluated.

Alcoholism is a sugar disorder.

Alcoholism is a sugar disorder. The sedating effects of alcohol are due to the alcohol itself. However, the craving for alcohol and its ability to cause liver disease both stem from its stimulation of fructose production, which then turns on the survival switch.

The observation that alcohol is another source of fructose also explains why drinking alcohol is associated with increased risk for metabolic syndrome, and especially increasing blood pressure and triglyceride levels. This is true for beer especially, as in addition to alcohol it also contains umami-rich brewer's yeast.

THE ORIGINS OF ALCOHOLISM

Alcoholism, like obesity and metabolic syndrome, also has its roots in evolution and the survival switch. As you may recall, during the mid-Miocene epoch, global cooling placed our ape ancestors in Europe and Asia at risk for starvation. Then, around 12 to 15 million years ago, the uricase mutation occurred, allowing those ancestors to generate more fat from the dwindling amount of fruit available to them. This helped those apes survive and allowed some of them to return to the African continent.

Unfortunately, volcanic activity and uplift had changed East Africa, and the apes had to pass through a much drier habitat of open savannas, where survival was still precarious. At the time, ripe fruit that had fallen on the ground and started to ferment was not edible, because our ancestors were not able to metabolize alcohol. This changed 10 million years ago, when a mutation occurred that

* For full disclosure, our group has a start-up company (Colorado Research Partners, LLC) that is developing inhibitors of fructose metabolism to block alcoholism. Most of the research and drug discovery has been supported by the National Institutes of Health.

increased our ability to metabolize alcohol fortyfold. This provided an additional survival advantage, as it allowed us to eat fermenting fruit and gave us another source of fructose: that produced by the polyol pathway when the alcohol we ingested triggered dehydration.

This mutation helped us survive a brutal time in history, but also gave us the gift, and the health consequences, of being able to drink alcohol.

BEHAVIORAL DISORDERS

As we've seen, when the survival switch is turned on in animals in the wild, it has multiple effects. It stimulates hunger and thirst, raises blood pressure, creates low-grade inflammation, and of course maximizes storage of fat. Another aspect of the switch is that it causes changes in behavior.

When a fasting animal runs out of fat, it must wake from its sleep or leave its nest and start foraging for food. If it does not find food, it will die—this is a desperate situation—and so the animal must be willing to enter new and unfamiliar areas in its search, which places it at risk from predators. Accordingly, it must be able to rapidly assess its environment, make fast decisions, and move quickly. There is no time for prolonged deliberation; the animal must be impulsive, for the longer it remains in an unfamiliar area, the more danger it is in. The animal cannot be timid, and if it runs into a predator, it may have to defend itself. Similarly, if it sees prey, it must attack even if there is a chance the prey might win. This cluster of behaviors—impulsivity, exploratory behavior, rapid decision-making, novelty-seeking, and risk-taking—is collectively referred to as the **foraging response**.

Fructose intake has been shown to trigger aspects of the foraging response. For example, a clinical study that compared the effects of drinking fructose versus glucose in healthy volunteers showed via MRI that, in comparison to glucose, fructose intake was associated with more immediate hunger and greater desire for high-calorie foods. Moreover, the area of the brain that controls willpower (that is, the prefrontal cortex) showed a decrease in electrical activity consistent with increased risk of giving in to temptation, decreased ability to say no, and a general decrease in willpower. These changes suggest fructose increases impulsivity, novelty-seeking, and risk-taking behaviors.

As you may recall, fructose metabolism results in the formation of uric acid, and there is evidence that uric acid stimulates the foraging response. For example, when blood uric acid levels are raised in laboratory rats, the animals initially become hyperactive. A study performed by Angelina Sutin at Florida State University reported that mice with high uric acid levels show stronger foraging behavior, including roaming over a greater area, being more excitable with spontaneous jumping, interacting more with novel objects presented to them, and showing more exploratory activity. Another study, led by Roy Cutler at the National Institutes of Health, confirmed that mice with high uric acid levels roamed much more widely over an open field than mice with normal levels, and showed more exploratory behavior. They also found that mice with higher uric acid levels had greater endurance on running wheels.*

That's mice. What about us? Dr. Sutin's research group also evaluated the relationship of blood uric acid levels with personality traits in humans, based on two different community studies. Again, a higher uric acid level was associated with characteristics of foraging behavior, including impulsivity, novelty-seeking, risk-taking, and decreased ability to deliberate (think before acting).

Many of these behaviors can be viewed, in some respects, as admirable. They are the same behaviors we use to characterize explorers, astronauts, and others willing to take great personal risks for potentially greater reward, both for themselves and for humankind. People with foraging personality types are the ones who break new ground, make scientific discoveries, start new industries, and open our world to new ideas.

Yet there is only a fine line separating the successful foraging response of the bold adventurer who guides us through the most perilous situations and the individual diagnosed with disorders such as attention deficit/hyperactivity disorder (ADHD), bipolar disorder, or mania due to impulsive, hyperactive, manic, and/or aggressive behavior. While I do not negate the role of genetics and other risk factors in these behavioral disorders, it is my belief that they

---

* While uric acid likely benefits endurance in the short-term as part of the foraging response, over time the negative effects of high uric acid appear to trump these effects.

represent a "hyperactive" foraging response stemming from excessive activation of the survival switch. Let us look at the evidence.

Attention Deficit/Hyperactivity Disorder

Attention deficit/hyperactivity disorder refers to a behavioral disorder in which an individual—child or adult—manifests behaviors such as fidgeting, inability to stay still, and excessive talking (hyperactivity) coupled with impulsivity, getting distracted easily, inattentiveness, and inability to focus or complete tasks (attention deficit). ADHD can affect school performance and the ability to sustain a job, and is also associated with increased risk of addiction.

Today, ADHD is extremely common. As of 2011, ADHD is reported to affect one in five high school boys and one in ten high school girls. Among children age four to seventeen, 11 percent have received the diagnosis. The condition often does not resolve with age, and many adults also show characteristics of ADHD. One survey found that one-third of households have someone in the family with ADHD.

Many factors likely play a role in causing ADHD, but I believe excessive intake of fructose may be an important one. For one thing, the prevalence of ADHD has increased dramatically in the last decades, in parallel with rising intake of sugar and HFCS—in fact, the frequency of ADHD is higher among people who are overweight or obese. A study of dietary patterns in seventeen different countries also found that impulsivity disorders such as ADHD, as well as anxiety and substance use disorders, are greatest in countries with high sugar intake.

Within-country studies also show that individuals with the highest sugar intake commonly have behavioral issues consistent with ADHD. For example, a study of tenth graders from Oslo, Norway, found that 50 percent of the boys and 20 percent of the girls drank at least one soft drink daily, and 10 percent of the boys drank four a day or more. When they were evaluated for hyperactivity and conduct problems, there was a direct relationship between such problems and drinking one or more sodas a day. Furthermore, children and adults with ADHD both have been reported to have higher uric acid levels. In one study of children between three and five years old, higher blood uric acid levels correlated with greater hyperactivity, shorter attention span, and less anger control.

In 2019, a French research group led by psychologist Charlotte Van den Driessche noted that individuals with ADHD do not simply show hyperactivity and impulsivity, but also show exploratory behavior whereby they can make rapid assessments consistent with what is required for successful foraging. This observation led her group to suggest that ADHD might itself be a manifestation of foraging behavior, as hyperactivity, exploratory behavior, and rapid assessment would all be useful behaviors in settings where food was scarce.

The idea that sugar is related to hyperactivity isn't new. Most parents and schoolteachers have been attributing children's hyperactive behavior to sugar consumption for decades. One study reported that 80 percent of elementary teachers believed sugar caused hyperactivity, and 40 percent thought that sugar had a role in causing ADHD. Many of you have probably witnessed children becoming hyperactive and manic within minutes of eating their Halloween candy (being on a "sugar high"), only to suddenly lose all their energy and "crash" an hour later. A recent study of Hispanic adolescents appeared to confirm this belief. In this study, children were given a high-sugar, low-fiber meal, and on a separate occasion a low-sugar, high-fiber meal. After the high-sugar meal, the children's activity increased markedly during the first three hours, then slowed down to below-normal levels. In contrast, after eating the low-sugar meal, their activity remained the same throughout the observation period.

Yet the medical literature calls a causal relationship between sugar and hyperactivity a myth. The reason is that a series of research studies, performed on children in the 1980s and early 1990s, could not demonstrate that sugar had any effect on hyperactivity or related behavioral issues. Most of these studies gave children sugar for a short period (from a single dose up to a daily dose for two or three weeks) and compared it to the effects of artificial sweeteners, such as aspartame or saccharin.

I believe these studies have several problems proving that sugar and hyperactivity are unrelated. First, they did not measure variations in uric acid levels. Our work suggests that the way fructose causes hyperactivity is by increasing uric acid. The rise typically occurs in the first hour after you eat fructose, which correlates with when the hyperactivity is commonly observed. However, the amount of uric acid produced can vary dramatically with how much sugar is eaten, how rapidly it is ingested, and whether the subject is accustomed to eating a lot of sugar. Furthermore, with long-term sugar intake, baseline uric acid levels remain high all day long, and so the normally acute change in uric acid in response to eating sugar is blunted. When this happens, a child (or adult) might have characteristics of hyperactivity or ADHD, but no longer show significant worsening of these symptoms after eating sugar. Since none of these prior studies measured the uric acid following sugar intake, they are hard to interpret.

A second problem is that these studies gave the children sucrose. As you know, sucrose contains both fructose and glucose. Although fructose causes foraging behavior, glucose does the opposite: it quells hunger and increases activity in the brain associated with enhanced willpower. While fructose-associated effects typically dominate the outcome when both fructose and glucose are given together, as in sucrose or HFCS, studies investigating the ability of sugar to cause ADHD should test not only table sugar, but also fructose alone, glucose alone,* and a low-glycemic carbohydrate.

Finally, most of the studies that failed to document sugar-induced hyperactivity compared diets high in sugar with diets containing an artificial sweetener rather than low-sugar diets. Artificial sweeteners may not be the right comparison, as these substances also stimulate a pleasure response in the brain but do not provide calories, and there is some evidence that this may cause dissatisfaction and agitation. Theoretically, agitation could mimic some signs associated with ADHD, like ability to concentrate or stay still, making it difficult to show differences between the two groups even if sucrose were causing signs of ADHD.

I admit, some of the evidence that high intake of fructose-containing sugars contributes to ADHD is based on associations, and we do need more direct clinical proof. Nevertheless, I feel there are good reasons to suspect that fructose may play a role.

Bipolar Disorder

Another behavioral disorder that I believe is caused partly by fructose is **bipolar disorder**, a condition characterized by episodes of mania followed by episodes of depression. Bipolar disorder is a common problem throughout the world, affecting 3 percent of individuals in the United States. The manic episodes may present with hyperactivity, talkativeness, racing thoughts, distractibility, and impulsiveness, and can also be associated with violent behavior. Indeed, some of the

---

* Even though, to add further confusion, some of the glucose would likely be converted to fructose in the body.

symptoms overlap with those of ADHD. In contrast, the episodes of depression can be severe, and are associated with uncontrollable feelings of sadness or hopelessness that can disrupt sleep and appetite and even lead to suicidal thoughts.

It seems possible to me that mania could, like ADHD, represent excessive foraging behavior in response to excess fructose-containing sugars or from the body's production of fructose. Bipolar disorder, too, has increased in parallel with the rise in sugar intake over the last fifty years. One study from the United States found that, between 1996 and 2004, the hospitalization rate for this disorder had increased sevenfold among children and 56 percent among adults. Another study, this one from Denmark, showed a modest doubling in the incidence of bipolar disorder in children between the late 1990s and 2014. While some of this increase may be due to increased awareness of the disorder and greater latitude in providing it as a diagnosis, the observation of increased hospitalization rates suggests a true increase in its frequency.

Researchers also have linked sugar intake with risk for bipolar disorder. For example, a study from New Zealand compared 89 adults that had been diagnosed with bipolar disorder with 445 age- and sex-matched individuals who did not have bipolar disorder. The subjects with bipolar disorder ingested much more sucrose and many more carbohydrates as part of their regular diet compared to the control group. Difference in intake of sugary beverages was especially significant, with the bipolar subjects drinking almost three a day compared to just one a day in the control group.

Subjects with bipolar disorder also frequently have elevated blood uric acid levels. An association between gout and mania was noted in the 1800s by Sir Alfred Baring Garrod, the physician who discovered that gout was caused by a high uric acid level. Uric acid levels tend to be higher in the manic phase. Lithium—the primary treatment for bipolar disease in the 1940s, and still in use today—was originally introduced as a means for treating gout, as it can reduce uric acid by enhancing its excretion in the urine. It was this use that led to the discovery that it could also help people with manic attacks. Since then, some scientists have surmised that uric acid might be involved in bipolar disorder, and this led to several trials, the goals of which were to determine if allopurinol (a drug that lowers uric acid levels) might be of benefit as an add-on therapy to lithium or other treatments for bipolar disorder. Interestingly, several of these trials showed benefit.

One particularly fascinating piece of evidence is the finding that individuals with bipolar disease make fructose in their brains. Specifically, studies of spinal fluid from these patients have found high levels of fructose, as well as sorbitol, the substance in the polyol pathway from which fructose is made. Fructose has also been found in postmortem brain tissue from patients with bipolar disorder, at higher levels than found in brains from individuals without this condition.

While it is relatively easily to speculate how fructose might contribute to mania given its ability to stimulate foraging responses, very little is known about how fructose may contribute to depression, or to the swinging back and forth between mania and depression that occurs in bipolar disorder. One might speculate that it relates to the changes in energy accompanying fluctuating ATP levels that occur with recurrent and high exposure to fructose. Clearly, we need more studies, especially when it comes to separating association from causation. However, the possibility that fructose may be contributing to bipolar disorder should be considered.

Aggression

Violent behavior often involves impulsivity, so the possibility that it sometimes might be triggered by excessive intake of fructose should not be dismissed.

Soft drink intake has been associated with violent behavior toward peers, family members, and intimate partners. For example, sugar intake in childhood has been linked to violent behavior in adulthood. In one study, 17,000 people were followed for more than twenty-five years, from age ten to thirty-five. Nearly 70 percent of those who developed violent behavior ate more than one sweet per day at age ten, compared to only about 40 percent of those that did not. Another study reported that drinking more than five soft drinks a week is associated with increased likelihood of carrying firearms. Similarly, elevated uric acid is associated with aggressive behavior. In one study of 106 individuals hospitalized following violent crimes, blood uric acid levels were significantly higher in those who committed the more violent acts compared to those who committed less violent offenses.

Of course, these studies show associations, and associations do not prove cause and effect. For example, it could be that both increased sugar intake and increased aggressive behavior are the result of socioeconomic status, as poverty has been linked to both. However, we can get some indirect evidence by going back to nature—specifically, by looking at ants. Within an ant colony, the worker ants are in charge of foraging expeditions, some traveling one hundred feet or more from the nest. They seek out and bring back to the colony honeydew (a sweet secretion containing sucrose, made by insects such as aphids) and nectar (also rich in sucrose), as well as insects (primarily a protein meal). However, forager ants themselves mainly eat sucrose, and experimental studies have shown that an ant's foraging activity and level of aggressiveness positively correlate with how much sugar it gets. In one study, ants were fed freeze-killed crickets and provided either regular water, water containing 2 percent sucrose, or water containing 20 percent sucrose. After twelve weeks, the ants fed 2 percent sucrose were more active than the ants on water, and more aggressive; they would threaten and sometimes attack other ants introduced into their living area. The ants that drank water containing 20 percent sucrose were also aggressive with the new arrivals, similar to those that received the lower dose of sucrose (though they were not any *more* aggressive, despite their higher sugar intake). One potential explanation is that the ants fed 20 percent sucrose gained a lot more fat than the other groups, resulting in them being less active—although they were still more active than the ants drinking water alone.*

As with the other behavioral disorders just discussed, we need more research into the potential contribution of fructose to aggressive behaviors. This feels especially urgent given the recent increase in mass shootings and violence in our schools and other public places—though, importantly, these events have multiple social, economic, and genetic causes, and solely blaming diet would be wrong.

COGNITION AND DEMENTIA

Another topic is whether fructose and persistent activation of the survival switch may affect cognition.

---

* The relationship between sugar and obesity in ants is not dissimilar to the one in mammals. For example, many ant species in northern latitudes shift from a protein-based diet of insects to sucrose in the fall, likely to help store fat for the winter. Likewise, ants living in the Sahara have extremely large fat stores, likely to provide water. Ants don't look fat, however, because it is all inside their exoskeleton!

One of the scariest diseases currently afflicting our society is Alzheimer's, the most common cause of dementia and now the sixth most common cause of death. Alzheimer's is an incapacitating disorder with no effective treatment. It is characterized by progressive death of neurons and brain shrinkage, along with formation of plaques rich in beta-amyloid (a specific type of protein) between neurons and accumulation of tau (another type of protein) within the neurons. The disease usually begins with loss of short-term memory, and progresses over a few years to full dementia.

Most scientists believe that the dementia could be prevented if we could find ways to block amyloid deposits or tau accumulation in the brain. However, several treatments that work by preventing or reducing amyloid plaques have failed, leading to questions of whether amyloid plaques are really the cause of the disease, and a search for other potential explanations.

Many scientists have noted that early Alzheimer's cases commonly display two notable characteristics. First, there are regions in the patient's brain where the uptake and metabolism of glucose is reduced, leading some to call Alzheimer's "brain diabetes" or "type 3 diabetes." Second, the energy factories in brain neurons are reduced in both number and function, leading to reduced ATP production. Both of these findings suggest the survival switch may be at work.

Indeed, risk factors for Alzheimer's disease include heavy intake of foods known to turn on the survival switch, such as sugar, high-glycemic carbohydrates, and salt. Conditions like obesity and diabetes are also associated with increased risk for Alzheimer's disease. If fructose is a root cause of obesity and diabetes, and they are associated with increased risk for Alzheimer's, it stands to reason that fructose should be suspect as a cause of Alzheimer's disease.

Experimental studies also support a link between sugar and cognition. For example, laboratory rats given sugary beverages show impaired thinking. One of my colleagues, physiologist Kieron Rooney, gave rats a 10 percent solution of sucrose, a concentration similar to a soft drink, for just two hours a day for a month. The rats that drank the sugary beverages had trouble finding their way through a maze. Even more alarmingly, this persisted for six weeks after the sugar was stopped. Similarly, children who drink a lot of soft drinks demonstrate worse performance in reading, writing, grammar, and math.

These studies suggest that intake of sugary beverages can have effects on cognition, and that these effects can persist. However, they do not necessarily mean that sucrose causes dementia. Even the finding that having one or more sugary beverages a day is associated with worse episodic memory (recollection of experiences or events in the past) and smaller brain volume is not conclusive.

However, there is increasing evidence linking fructose with Alzheimer's. The brains of Alzheimer's patients show elevated fructose levels, with amounts four to six times higher than those found in brains from individuals of similar age and sex who did not have Alzheimer's. The highest elevations were found in regions classically affected by the disease. There is also evidence that much of this fructose is being made in the brain via the polyol pathway. As in bipolar disorder, high amounts of sorbitol, the precursor to fructose, have also been found. As we know, once fructose is produced, it triggers the survival switch, decreasing the amount of ATP in the cells. Additionally, levels of the enzyme responsible for "sweeping up" AMP, which would otherwise be made back into ATP to sustain energy levels, are approximately twofold higher in the brains of Alzheimer's patients, compared to age-matched controls.

I believe the way fructose leads to Alzheimer's is as follows. You may recall that activation of the survival switch protects the brain in the event that there is no food available, and that it does so by preventing the uptake of glucose from the blood into the muscle and liver, thereby reserving the glucose so it can be used by the brain. The switch does this by blocking the effects of insulin, as muscle and liver cells need insulin to absorb and use glucose, whereas much of the brain does not. There are exceptions, however: the brain regions associated with memory and decision-making *do* require insulin for glucose uptake.* Studies by Fernando Gomez-Pinilla, a neurophysiologist from UCLA, showed that rats ingesting fructose lose their responsiveness to insulin in these areas of the brain, resulting in less uptake of glucose. In effect, fructose may be causing resistance to the effects of insulin not only in the muscle and liver (what we call systemic insulin resistance or

Fructose may be causing resistance to the effects of insulin not only in the muscle and liver, but also in the brain, and it is this that may be the root cause of Alzheimer's disease.

---

* If you're curious, the specific regions include the hippocampus, striatum, hypothalamus, and the sensorineural cortex.

prediabetes), but also in key regions of the brain associated with memory, and it is this that may be the root cause of Alzheimer's disease.

But what survival benefit would restricting glucose to those specific areas of the brain confer? As we've seen, impulsivity and exploratory behavior are foraging behaviors. An animal with impaired memory might be more willing to explore dangerous areas (because they do not remember the potential dangers they might encounter), and one with impaired decision-making might be more impulsive. So it stands to reason that fructose's ability to boost foraging by causing insulin resistance in these regions of the brain is a survival response.

Initially, the short-term inhibition of function in these regions, resulting from activation of the survival switch, would provide a survival advantage, but with recurrent or chronic stimulation, it could lead to brain damage. Chronically reducing glucose uptake to these valuable neurons could eventually starve them and impair their function. This would be amplified by the oxidative stress that fructose metabolism causes to the mitochondria, and the attendant reduction in ATP production. Once ATP levels get low enough, the neuron dies. Alzheimer's is the result. According to this viewpoint, the subsequent changes to the brains of Alzheimer's patients, such as amyloid and tau protein accumulation, are secondary, and the primary underlying cause of Alzheimer's is chronic activation of the survival switch.

The Uric Acid Paradoxes

If fructose metabolism does play a role in Alzheimer's disease, it is reasonable to think that elevated uric acid should also be a risk factor, as it is a product of fructose metabolism. In support of this idea, both a study in Taiwan and a US study evaluating Medicare claims found that people who take medications to lower uric acid have significantly lower risk of developing dementia.

There are some who believe uric acid does not predict dementia, but rather genius and achievement. A 1955 letter written by metallurgist and physicist Egon Orowan to the journal *Science* noted that uric acid is very similar to caffeine in chemical structure and that it might act as a stimulant for the brain. Orowan proposed that the reason humans are so advanced compared to other species is that we lost the uricase gene; the higher uric acid levels that resulted, he suggested, may have beneficial effects on brain function. There is also anecdotal evidence that many outstanding individuals suffered from gout, including explorers (Christopher Columbus), rulers (Alexander the Great, Queen Victoria), artists (Michelangelo, Peter Paul Rubens), composers (Ludwig van Beethoven), authors (Charles Dickens, Goethe), inventors (Benjamin Franklin, Leonardo da Vinci), and scientists (Isaac Newton, Galileo). Observations such as this led to several studies of whether higher uric acid levels are associated with higher intelligence. All of the studies had negative findings—having higher uric acid levels does not mean you are smarter.

However, some studies did suggest that people with high uric acid levels tend to do better on exams and are high achievers (note that intelligence and achievement are different beasts). In one study, high school students in the top quarter of their class were found to have significantly higher uric acid levels than the rest of the students; they achieved higher grades than expected for their IQ and were more likely to go to college. They also tended to be more confident, to date more, and to spend more time doing leisure activities. In another study of over fifty university professors, in which an extensive evaluation system was used to assess drive, achievement, and leadership, higher uric acid levels were a strong predictor for these characteristics independent of alcohol, caffeine, hours of sleep, and body weight. Other studies also support the idea that a high uric acid level may indicate one's likelihood to become a high achiever, though a few found no statistically significant associations.

While this may appear to be a paradox, I suspect the association of uric acid with achievement on the one hand and dementia on the other might reflect the extent to which the survival switch is turned on, as well as the duration. Some features of foraging behavior, like rapid response time, openness, and modest risk-taking, could be beneficial in the classroom and predictive of success. Exploratory behavior and novelty-seeking may boost creativity. However, over time these behaviors could progress to more of a dysfunctional state such as ADHD or a disease such as Alzheimer's. I would therefore not view having elevated blood uric acid levels as an advantage, at least in the long term.

Another paradox is that, while subjects with high uric acid levels are at greater risk for developing dementia, when people present with dementia, their uric acid levels are often low. This is a little easier to understand, as numerous studies have shown that Alzheimer's patients often lose substantial weight in the months before they are diagnosed. Since the concentration of uric acid in the blood is largely driven by food intake, it is to be expected that these patients' uric acid levels would be low at the time of diagnosis.

There is one final uric acid paradox to consider. While an elevated uric acid level predicts strokes and dementia, there is some counterintuitive evidence that, when a stroke occurs, administering uric acid may help limit the extent of the stroke. This suggests that uric acid can be beneficial during times of crisis. Some studies suggest that uric acid may block oxidative stress in the areas of the stroke. (Uric acid is a unique molecule, as it blocks oxidative stress when outside the cell, despite causing oxidative stress inside it.) However, based on my studies of uric acid, I suspect that its benefits more likely arise from its role in stimulating protective features of the survival switch, such as reducing brain cells' need for oxygen.

There is increasing interest of late in the role of fructose, carbohydrates, and uric acid in the brain. One leader in this area is David Perlmutter, a respected neurologist and author of *Grain Brain* and *Drop Acid*, who has written extensively on how carbohydrates and sugar may have a role in dementia, as well as on the effects of fructose and uric acid. Another is William Wilson, a family physician who is convinced from years of clinical practice that sugary foods and high-glycemic carbohydrates are contributing to many behavioral disorders, including depression, ADHD, and anxiety disorders, which he collectively ascribes to "CARB syndrome" (Carbohydrate-Associated Reversible Brain syndrome).* Wilson is convinced that reducing the intake of sugary foods (those that contain fructose) and high-glycemic carbohydrates (those that can produce fructose) can result in improvements in these disorders. The next step would be to perform clinical trials to see if he is right.

From these last two chapters, a clear pattern emerges. Whereas engagement of the survival switch is of benefit during times of temporary crisis, when it is engaged chronically or excessively, it can lead to medical problems. As long as we ate a diet that only included fruits and occasional honey, especially seasonally, we were unlikely to develop persistent obesity or its partner diseases. We got into trouble when we switched our diet to one that is both high in foods

---

* Wilson's website, if you're interested in learning more, is carbsyndrome.com.

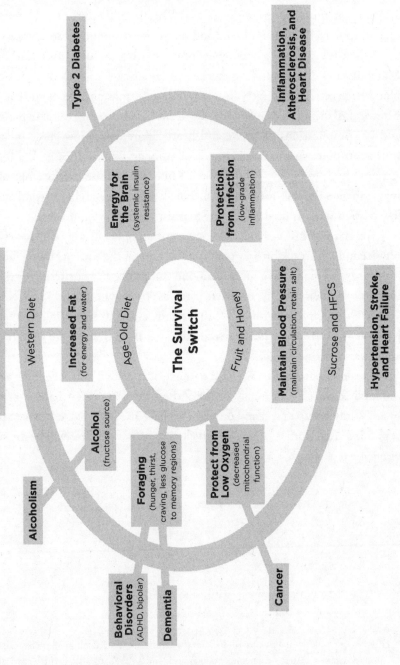

that activate the survival switch (such as sugar, high-glycemic carbs, and salt) and has year-round access to these foods. This has allowed the switch to be kept on and spurred the rise in obesity and many noncommunicable diseases.

When the survival switch goes into overdrive, we don't just gain weight. Many diseases also result. The increase in fat storage leads to obesity, elevated blood triglycerides, and fatty liver, while insulin resistance leads to type 2 diabetes and Alzheimer's disease. The effects on blood pressure cause hypertension and its complications of stroke and heart failure, while low-grade inflammation contributes to the development of coronary artery disease. The foraging response leads to behavioral disorders, while the fructose produced by alcohol may enhance the risk for addiction. Finally, fructose's ability to protect us in low-oxygen states is used by tumors to assist their growth and spread.

Today, these diseases are the most common ones affecting our society. As a physician, I am struck by how common they are in the patients filling our medical wards. So many have more than one condition that our residents describe the typical patient as a list of letters (such as "51yo with DM, HTN, NAFLD, CAD, CVA, admitted with MI"*) that might sound like a foreign language but is everyday parlance for us. Few recognize that these diseases are all part of one epidemic with one root cause.

The good news is that we have strong evidence that persistent activation of the survival switch is a primary driver of these diseases, and—thanks to research by my study group and many others—we have the knowledge we need to prevent this switch from turning on, as well as to turn it off. This will be the subject of our final chapters.

---

* Fifty-one-year-old with a history of diabetes, hypertension, non-alcoholic fatty liver disease, coronary artery disease, and cerebral vascular accident (stroke), admitted with a myocardial infarction (heart attack).

PART III

Outfoxing
Nature

CHAPTER 8

Understanding Sugar in Our Diet

As a society, we eat a lot of sugar. One study of over 85,000 packaged foods showed that 68 percent of them contained fructose, glucose, or combined fructose-glucose caloric sweeteners. Indeed, over 77 percent of all the foods we eat contain caloric sweeteners. According to the American Heart Association, the average person takes in the equivalent of twenty-two teaspoons of added sugars, specifically, a day, accounting for 15 to 20 percent of their overall caloric intake. Disadvantaged and minority populations tend to ingest even more (likely due to the lower cost of packaged foods high in added sugars, as we saw), as do adolescents and young adults. For some individuals, a quarter or more of their diet is added sugars.

Many medical societies recommend reducing intake of added sugars. The American Heart Association counsels that women ingest no more than six teaspoons (25 grams or 100 calories) of high-fructose corn syrup and sucrose a day and that men ingest no more than nine (37 grams or 150 calories). The World Health Organization recommendation is even stronger. They suggest that the ideal goal is to reduce both added and natural sugars, such as in honey and fruit juices, to less than 5 percent of all calories (about 7 teaspoons for a man eating 2,200 calories a day). These and other recommendations by the medical and public health communities have been accompanied by political attempts to reduce sugar intake by taxation, or by removing sugary beverages from schools, and a more general attempt to educate the public. To some extent, these approaches are working. Soft drink intake, for example, has progressively decreased since 2005. Yet it is clear we have a long way to go.

Given the importance of reducing fructose intake for our overall health, it's important to review the forms it takes, and how to recognize it in our foods. However, the broader goal of this chapter is to learn from the science how to minimize the effects on our bodies of the fructose we eat, and to resolve some questions, misconceptions, and controversies in the literature about sugar.

TYPES OF SUGAR, AND READING NUTRITION LABELS

The first step to reducing the amount of sugar we eat is being able to identify how much of it we are ingesting now. This begins with being able to recognize and understand the different types of sugars added to foods. So let's start with some general guidelines for doing so.

Almost all sugars can cause obesity. These include the sugars that only contain fructose, those that contain fructose and glucose, and those that only contain glucose (which can be converted to fructose in the body), as we've learned. There is one exception: dairy-based sugars, such as lactose, the principal sugar in milk. Lactose lacks fructose, and while it does contain glucose (along with another sugar, galactose), it does not appear to increase the risk for obesity.

The US Food and Drug Administration (FDA) has recently changed the "Nutrition Facts" labels to include both **total sugars** and **added sugars** in each serving of food. Total sugars include all of the sugars present in a food, which can include healthy sugars such as lactose in milk, so it is most important to look at the amount of added sugars. Added sugars are given both in grams and as a percentage of daily recommended upper limits, which the FDA currently defines as 50 grams (200 calories), or 10 percent of an average daily diet of 2,000 calories. However, sugars from fruit juices or concentrates in fruit jams and jellies, sauces (such as applesauce), or pure fruit juice, and the sugars present in honey, are not included in added sugars. So, when it comes to foods containing honey or fruit concentrates, you should also look at total sugar content.

While looking at added sugar content is a quick and easy way to determine how much HFCS and sucrose are present in a particular food, it is also helpful to know the various names for the many sugars we eat and what types of sugars they represent. For example, there are many different types of (and names for) sucrose (table sugar), including refined sucrose (powdered sugar, crystalline sugar, granulated sugar, confectioner's sugar, baker's sugar, icing sugar, caster sugar), partially purified sucrose (caramel, brown sugar, molasses, treacle, muscovado, turbinado, demerara, raw sugar, sugarcane juice, panocha, panella, piloncillo), and sucrose from other sources (maple sugar, palm sugar, date sugar, sorghum syrup, coconut sugar). Sucrose is also sometimes referred to as saccharose.

There has been some discussion that less-purified sugars, such as brown sugar, may be healthier, as some argue that these sugars might contain substances that could lessen the effects of the sugar. However, minimal evidence supports this, so I recommend considering all forms of sucrose as equal in biologic effects, and equally worth reducing.

Different Types of Sugars			
Fructose	Fructose-Glucose Combinations	Glucose and High-Glycemic Sugars	Dairy-Based Sugars
Fruit sugar	Sucrose (table sugar)	Dextrose (glucose)	Milk sugar (lactose)
Dried fruits	High-fructose corn syrup (HFCS)	Corn syrup	Galactose
Fruit juices	Invert sugar	Rice syrup	
Agave nectar/syrup		Brown rice syrup	
Honey		Maltose	
		Malt sugar	
		Maltotroise	
		Barley malt syrup	
		Trehalose	

Note that the foods listed as containing only fructose also contain small amounts of other sugars, such as sucrose and glucose.

Knowing the sugar content of various foods is a good start, but there is much more that we can do to minimize the amount of fructose we eat, and its effects on our body, besides simply looking at food labels and choosing foods with less added sugar. Let's dive in to better understand the particular nuances of fructose: how we can use the science we have learned to make wise decisions on the types of sugar we should eat, and how best we should eat them.

QUESTION 1.
DO WE NEED TO CONSIDER THE AMOUNTS OF SUGAR (AND ESPECIALLY FRUCTOSE) IN FRUITS AND VEGETABLES?

These foods are widely viewed as healthy and often recommended, but many of these foods contain fructose (yes, vegetables, too!). Furthermore, many animals eat fruit to activate the survival switch. On the surface, this suggests that fruit in particular might be especially bad.

To get to the answer, we need to look closer at the biology of how fructose activates the survival switch.

When it comes to gaining weight from fructose, the liver is where the action happens. When the switch is activated in the liver, it drives all aspects of metabolic syndrome, including abdominal fat accumulation, prediabetes, and fatty liver. As we learned previously, the liver does not control our craving for sugar, which appears to be related more to metabolism of fructose in the brain and intestines. However, when it comes to weight gain and the rest of the survival switch's negative health effects, the liver is key.

We know the liver is the grand conductor because our research group performed studies in which we specifically blocked fructokinase, the enzyme that metabolizes fructose, only in the liver. What we found was that, if we got rid of fructokinase in the liver, animals that were fed fructose were completely protected from weight gain, for they compensated for the fructose they drank by eating less food. The fructose did not cause hunger, as it normally would have, and the animals did not develop leptin resistance, so weight gain did not occur. The mice also did not accumulate fat in their adipose tissues or their livers, and they did not become prediabetic.

What this means is that to prevent obesity and metabolic syndrome, we need to minimize the amount of fructose metabolized in the liver. This is important when we consider the amount of fructose in our foods. Less fructose ingested means less fructose metabolized in our liver. But there is a twist.

Whenever we eat fructose, a small amount is metabolized in the intestine before it can reach the liver. This portion, which is in the 4- to 5-gram range, is metabolized like any other calorie—and notably, it does not activate the switch. In effect, the intestine acts as a shield. This means we do not have to worry about eating foods with only small amounts of fructose, such as carrots, sweet peas, pumpkins, and other vegetables.

To prevent obesity and metabolic syndrome, we need to minimize the amount of fructose metabolized in the liver.

Fruits are a little different from vegetables. They tend to include more fructose per serving, so while much of the fructose may be removed by the intestines, some still gets to the liver, especially for fruits that contain 8 grams of fructose or more (see the table on the next page). However, whole fruits contain substances that tend to block the effects of fructose, such as vitamin C,* plant compounds known as **flavonoids**,† potassium,‡ and fiber. Kiwi, for example, is low in fructose and high in vitamin C. Blueberries and strawberries are especially high in flavonoids. Cherries contain additional substances that can lower uric acid. Many fruits, as well as vegetables, are also rich in soluble fiber, which can reduce or slow the absorption of fructose, and therefore reduce or slow its metabolism.

Still, I recommend limiting intake of fruits with high fructose content (>8 g/serving), perhaps by having only a half-serving at a time, and instead choosing fruits with lower fructose content. I would eat figs sparingly, for they have the highest fructose content of all fruits, with one cup having the same amount of fructose as a 12-ounce soft drink. (Recall the role played by the fig,

---

* Which, as we saw in chapter four, protects the energy factories from oxidative stress resulting from the metabolism of fructose. Vitamin C also stimulates the excretion of uric acid in the urine.

† Some of which may have medicinal properties, and which provide other health benefits, including blocking oxidative stress.

‡ We found that potassium, like vitamin C, can block some of the effects of the survival switch. However, the goal with potassium is to keep levels in the normal range, as both low and high levels of potassium in the blood can affect heart rhythm. Do not take potassium supplements without discussing with your physician.

and its disappearance, in the lives of our early ancestors. Figs have been widely beloved in history as a survival food; for example, some nomadic Bedouins would wear "fig strings" around their neck when crossing the desert.)

Most dried fruits should be viewed as similar to candy, and also eaten only sparingly. They are rich in fructose, and the process of drying them can destroy many of the nutrients present in fresh fruits that blunt fructose's effects. Fresh cranberries, for example, have little fructose when picked from a vine, but one-third of a cup of dried cranberries may contain up to 25 grams of sugar. And, of course, many are sold with added sugar to blunt their tartness.

Natural Fruits		
High Fructose Content (>8g fructose/serving)	Medium Fructose Content (4–8g fructose/serving)	Low Fructose Content (<4g fructose/serving)
Dried figs (1 cup) 23g	Medjool date (1) 7.8g	Strawberries (1 cup) 3.8g
Dried apricot (1 cup) 16g	Blueberries (1 cup) 7.4g	Cherries (1 cup) 3.8g
Mango (half) 16g	Banana 7g	Star fruit 3.6g
Green or red grapes (1 cup) 12g	Honeydew melon (one-eighth) 7g	Blackberries (1 cup) 3.5g
Raisins (1/4 cup) 12g	Papaya (half) 6g	Kiwi 3.4g
Pear 12g	Orange 6g	Clementine 3.4g
Watermelon (1 slice) 11g	Peach 6g	Raspberries (1 cup) 3.0g
Persimmon 11g	Nectarine 5g	Cantaloupe (one-eighth) 2.8g
Apple 9.5g	Tangerine 5g	Plum 2.6g
	Boysenberries (1 cup) 5g	Deglet noor date 2.6g
	Grapefruit (half) 4g	Apricot 1.3g
	Pineapple (1 slice) 4g	Guava 1.2g
		Prune 1.2g
		Cranberries (1 cup) 0.7g
		Lemon 0.6g
		Lime 0g
A serving consists of the specified amount or refers to an individual fruit.		

There is a difference between how we eat fruit and how animals that are trying to activate the survival switch eat fruit. Animals in the wild prefer ripe fruit, and recall that when fruit ripens, the fructose content increases while the vitamin C content falls. We tend to like tart fruit. Also, most of us will only eat one or two fruit, or one or two servings of a fruit, at one time. Animals will eat many fruit at a time, giving them a much larger fructose load. For example, a grizzly bear may eat one hundred thousand buffalo berries in one day—a few more than you or I would.

We evaluated the role of fruits with Magdalena Madero, chief of nephrology at the National Institute of Cardiology Ignacio Chávez in Mexico City. She conducted a clinical trial where she gave a low-fructose diet to two groups of overweight and obese women to see if it would affect weight loss. While both groups were restricted from soft drinks, fruit juices, and sugary foods and placed on mild calorie restriction, one group was allowed to eat whole fruits. As such, this latter group tended to have a moderate intake of fructose. At the end of the study, both groups had lost weight (the group whose diets included fruits actually showed greater weight loss!) and showed similar improvements in the features of metabolic syndrome. We believe that, for the group with moderate fructose intake, the benefits of whole fruit (vitamin C, flavonoids, potassium, and fiber) outweighed the risks from the small amounts of fructose they contained.

Although whole fruits are something we should include in our diet, I recommend limiting fruit juices, smoothies, and fruit drinks. Each of these drinks typically contains several fruits, so their overall fructose content is higher. The process of making fruit juice also removes much of the fiber. And studies suggest that both fruit drinks (to which sugar is often added) and, to a lesser extent, natural fruit juices increase the risk for obesity and diabetes. This is particularly true for children, a finding that led the American Pediatric Society to recommend that children under age six should drink no more than 6 ounces of juice a day, and older children no more than 8 to 12 ounces per day. Personally, I would limit this even more.

Takeaway: Consider vegetables fructose free. Eat fresh fruits, but limit the total fructose of the fruit you consume in a given meal or snack to 8 grams. Dried fruits, processed foods containing fruits, fruit-based jams and jellies, and juices can contain a lot of fructose. While an apple a day keeps the doctor away, five apples a day and the doctor you'll pay.

QUESTION 2.
IS THERE ANY DIFFERENCE BETWEEN CONSUMING ADDED SUGARS IN DRINKS AND EATING ADDED SUGARS IN FOOD?

In other words, what is the difference between eating jelly beans that have 20 grams of HFCS and drinking a soda with 20 grams of HFCS?

If activating the survival switch were simply a matter of calories, then the effect of HFCS would be the same whether you ate it in jelly beans or drank it in a soda. Unfortunately, this is not the case. Drinking sugar is often much worse than eating it. Why might that be?

The survival switch is triggered by a fall in ATP levels in the liver, so what matters most is how much fructose gets to the liver. If the liver receives a large load of fructose, then the fall in ATP is severe and the switch is thrown into high gear. If only a small load of fructose reaches the liver, the metabolic effects are milder. This means that, despite the fact that we have been speaking of this process as controlled by a simple on/off switch, it is really more of a dimmer, which can initiate an intense or mild response depending on the situation.

In other words, the liver is responding to the *concentration* of fructose it receives, not the amount. If the fructose trickles in slowly, the concentration of fructose to which the liver is exposed will be lower than if all of the fructose arrives at once.

Drinking sugar is often much worse than eating it, because the liver responds to the concentration *of fructose it receives, not the amount.*

This is the reason soft drinks activate the switch much more easily than solid sugar. Soft drinks contain a lot of sugar (for example, a 20-ounce soda contains about 17 teaspoons of HFCS, 9 teaspoons of which are fructose). Soft drinks are also commonly drunk in just a few minutes and, because they are liquid, require minimal digestion. This results in a rapid flooding of the liver with both fructose and glucose. In contrast, solid foods have to be digested and so take more time to reach the liver. (This is one reason whole fruits do not tend to activate the switch: the fiber in them helps slows absorption.) As a consequence, the fructose in solid foods reaches the liver more slowly, and the switch is not turned on as strongly.

An experimental study performed by nutritionist and geneticist John Speakman confirmed that mice given liquid sugar become much more obese than mice fed solid sugar. Clinical studies have also compared intake of liquid sugar (from soft drinks or other beverages) with intake of solid sugars (from sweets and desserts) in humans, and in every case there was evidence that liquid sugar is more likely to cause obesity and/or prediabetes. In one study, young adults were randomly selected to either drink one 8-ounce soft drink per day or eat jelly beans with equivalent sugar content for four weeks. After a four-week "washout" period in which they went back to their regular diets, the groups switched: those assigned to the soft drinks instead ate jelly beans, and vice versa, for another four weeks. At the end of the eight weeks, the researchers found that when subjects *drank* the sugar, they ate around 17 percent more calories than when they were eating jelly beans. After four weeks of soft drinks, subjects weighed more and had more fat. In contrast, no weight gain occurred during the four weeks they ate jelly beans.

While liquid sugar is more likely to cause obesity than solid sugar, how fast you drink the liquid sugar also makes a difference. To demonstrate this, our collaborator Mehmet Kanbay at Koç University in Istanbul gave volunteers apple juice, which has a fructose content similar to soft drinks. Half of the group drank 500 mL (equal to about 17 ounces) in five minutes, while the other half drank 125 mL every fifteen minutes for one hour. At the end of the hour, both groups had drunk the *same amount* of apple juice, but the differences between them were striking. Those who drank the apple juice quickly experienced a rapid increase in uric acid and vasopressin, the fat hormone. In contrast, changes were milder in the subjects who spread the apple juice out over an hour. Since the rise in uric acid and vasopressin represents evidence that the survival switch has been activated, the implication is that, when it comes to soft drinks, if you must drink them, slow is safer than fast.

Several years ago, there was a proposal to tax soft drinks in New York City due to their high sugar content. The soft drink industry argued that it was unfair to single out soft drinks when other foods also contained high amounts of sugar, and in part because of this argument, the beverage tax did not pass. We now know the industry's argument is flawed.

There is one more conclusion we might draw from this work, which is that it may be possible to "have your cake and eat it, too." That is, if you eat a sugar-rich dessert slowly enough, it might be possible to avoid triggering the survival switch. The cake would just be calories. (The problem, of course, is that it is almost impossible to eat a dessert slowly!) The same would be true for sipping a soft drink slowly, over an hour, as opposed to drinking it rapidly. This is also why drinking a soft drink may be worse if ingested alone as opposed to during a meal: mixing liquid sugar with food slows its absorption.

> **Takeaway:** Liquid sugar is a bigger culprit than solid sugar, and guzzling down a soft drink is the most powerful way to activate the survival switch. Avoid all sugary soft drinks, energy drinks, fruit juice, and sugary teas and coffee. If you must indulge, drink slowly and be sure to pair with food.

QUESTION 3.
IS THERE A REASON IT FELT AS IF I COULD EAT SUGAR WITH IMPUNITY WHEN I WAS YOUNG, AND NOW IT SEEMS SO EASY TO GAIN WEIGHT FROM ALMOST ANYTHING I EAT?

You aren't imagining it! It does become easier to gain weight as we get older. There are likely multiple reasons for this, and one of the more important reasons is a change in our body metabolism, which we will discuss further in chapter ten. However, there is another reason: the more we eat fructose, the more efficient at absorbing and metabolizing fructose we become.

As we know, when we eat sucrose, it breaks down to fructose and glucose in the gut. Both sugars are then absorbed separately in the intestine and eventually transported to the liver. Evidence suggests that the presence of glucose can assist the absorption of fructose, and vice versa. However, when fructose is given alone, absorption is quite limited, and some fructose frequently lingers in the gut and is passed into the stool—something we see frequently in infants and children. However, the more fructose we ingest (whether as pure fructose or as sucrose or HFCS), the easier it becomes for us to absorb and metabolize fructose the next time we are exposed.

The same is true for our ability to make fructose: the more fructose we make, the better we become at it. Normally the liver makes very little fructose, as the polyol pathway that produces it is minimally present. However, if this pathway is recurrently stimulated—say, if the liver is bathed with high concentrations of glucose from high-glycemic foods—this changes. Over time, the body starts to make fructose more and more easily from these high-glycemic carbohydrates. A similar process can occur with salty foods, umami foods, and fructose itself: the more these foods stimulate the polyol pathway, the easier it becomes for us to generate fructose from the foods many of us commonly eat.

The ability of chronic fructose exposure to accelerate the production, absorption, and metabolism of fructose is a powerful amplifying system that makes us fatter over time. To demonstrate this, Gaby Sánchez-Lozada, a physiologist from the National Cardiology Institute in Mexico City, gave laboratory rats either regular drinking water or water containing fructose for two weeks. During that time, the animals that received fructose became more sensitive to fructose and increased their ability both to absorb and metabolize it. She then took the fructose water away from that second group of rats, so that all the rats were on the same diet overnight, before giving both groups the equivalent of a large soft drink. The rats that had been previously exposed to fructose had a massive response. They showed a huge fall in ATP in their livers, consistent with marked activation of the survival switch; their blood and liver fats rose, as did uric acid levels; and they had increased oxidative stress in the liver. In contrast, the rats that had not received fructose for the first two weeks had a much more modest response to the soft drink.

The potential clinical relevance of these findings was demonstrated in a study we performed with Jillian Sullivan and Shikha Sundaram, pediatric specialists who often treat children with fatty liver disease and obesity. We compared how well fructose was absorbed and metabolized in lean children, children with obesity, and children with obesity who had fatty liver, and the findings were striking. The lean children did not absorb the fructose very well and metabolized it slowly. In contrast, the obese children absorbed fructose much more easily, and the children who were both obese and had fatty liver absorbed and metabolized fructose to an even greater extent. While other explanations are possible, the observation that obesity and fatty liver correlate with ease of fructose absorption and metabolism supports the idea that higher past exposure to fructose-containing sugars makes us more susceptible to fructose's effects.

This increased fructose sensitivity from greater exposure may partially explain why we are resistant to the effects of fructose when we are young, but over time become more likely to activate the switch. It may also explain why some individuals who have a history of eating a lot of added sugars may not see a lot of weight loss after reducing sugar, as even low doses of sugar may be able to activate their survival switch. Further, it may be an additional reason many animals gorge on fruit ahead of hibernation: the more they eat, the more efficient they get at absorbing and metabolizing the fructose, and the better they get at putting on fat.

The good news is that there's an easy fix. This increased sensitivity can be reversed by eliminating fructose from your diet for five days to two weeks. Studies in animals show that animals will rapidly reset their system when fructose is removed from their diet. In humans, this is likely why the severe two-week restriction in carbohydrates that is commonly recommended when starting a low-carb diet is so important: it allows the body to revert to its original settings, something I call "rebooting the system."

> **Takeaway:** The more fructose we eat, the more sensitive we become to its effects. In other words, the more you like sugar, the more sugar likes you. Fortunately, you can "reboot" your system with short-term carbohydrate restriction.

QUESTION 4.
ARE ARTIFICIAL SWEETENERS SAFE?
WILL USING THEM HELP ME LOSE WEIGHT?

Artificial sweeteners contain minimal calories and are typically used as a substitute for sucrose or HFCS, creating drinks or foods that taste sweet but are lower in calories. The name "nonnutritive sweeteners" is sometimes preferred over "artificial sweeteners" because some of the sweeteners are derived from natural products. The most common artificial sweeteners on the market include saccharin, aspartame, stevia, and sucralose, but there are others as well (see the table below).

Despite having minimal calories, *some* artificial sugars still activate the survival switch. For example, sorbitol, which is often used in sugar-free syrups, is part of the polyol pathway and is actually converted to fructose in the body. Absorption of sorbitol is variable, but it can be significant. Tagatose is another artificial sugar that can substitute for fructose and directly activates the survival switch because it, like fructose, is metabolized by fructokinase. While saccharin does not activate the survival switch, it has been reported to cause insulin resistance in animals, likely through an effect on gut bacteria. Excess intake of saccharin in mice has also led to bladder tumors. My recommendation is to avoid these three sweeteners.

I am also not a big fan of aspartame and advantame, which are chemically related to each other. When the body breaks down these sweeteners, one of their by-products is methanol, which is toxic. There are anecdotal reports that ingestion of aspartame can be associated with headaches, difficulty concentrating, agitation, and even impaired memory in humans. Laboratory rats fed aspartame also have trouble remembering how to get through a maze. (This might explain why clinical trials performed in the 1980s failed to show a difference between sucrose and aspartame in causing symptoms of ADHD, as described in chapter seven.)

Artificial Sweeteners (Nonnutritive Sweeteners)			
Synthetic Compounds	Natural Compounds	Sugar Alcohols	Chemically Similar to Fructose
Saccharin (Sweet'N Low)*	Stevia (Truvia)	Sorbitol**	Allulose
Aspartame (Equal, Nutrasweet)	Monk fruit	Xylitol	Yacon syrup**
Sucralose (Splenda)	Invert sugar	Maltitol	Tagatose**
Acesulfame (AceK)		Erythritol	
Advantame			
*May cause insulin resistance through effects on gut bacteria. **May be converted to fructose or act like fructose in the body.			

In terms of the other sweeteners, my family tends to use sucralose or stevia. Sucralose has a sweet taste and contains minimal calories. It's a sugar to which chlorine has been added, and its use is controversial; some experts have voiced concerns that it has not been adequately tested. However, those studies that have been performed have not identified any concerns. Stevia is a commonly used sweetener, preferred by some as it is a natural product derived from the stevia plant native to Brazil. The one downside is that stevia—as well as another natural sweetener, monk fruit—can have a slightly bitter aftertaste. I also like the sugar alcohols (other than sorbitol), and especially maltitol, which is often added to carbohydrate-free ice creams. However, sugar alcohols can cause abdominal bloating and diarrhea for some, especially if one's serving size is large.

Yacon syrup is an interesting sweetener, as it consists of a chain of fructose molecules called **fructans**. Humans cannot break fructans down to generate fructose, but some bacteria can, and people harboring those bacteria in their gut could theoretically convert fructans present in yacon syrup, as well as other foods such as wheat and onions, into fructose that could then be absorbed. The amount is relatively small, but if yacon syrup became your principal sweetener, it could become an issue.*

The most recent addition to the sweetener lineup is allulose. Allulose is chemically similar to fructose but, unlike fructose, does not activate the survival switch, and thus may be a good choice. However, while most artificial sweeteners are much sweeter than sucrose and so can be used in small amounts, allulose is less sweet than sucrose, and therefore larger amounts are needed to achieve the same level of sweetness. Much of the sweetener is excreted in the urine, and its potential long-term effects on the kidney and bladder are not well known. I would view this sweetener with cautious optimism.

---

* Interestingly, the bacteria that cause dental cavities live off the fructose we eat as their main energy source, storing the extra fructose as fructans in the crevices of our teeth, which they then dine on when we are not actively ingesting food. Fructans can also contribute to disease in horses, which use gut bacteria to convert fructans in rich pasture grass into fructose. In a collaboration with Tanja Hess from Colorado State University, we found evidence that fructose produced from fructans in grass may be responsible for both equine metabolic syndrome as well as founder, a disabling arthritis that is a major disease in racehorses. Victims of founder include Secretariat, the Triple Crown winner.

So the answer to the first question is that, while we can never be fully certain, some artificial sweeteners appear to be safe. But do they protect people from gaining weight? Essentially every study on the subject has shown that substituting drinks with artificial sugars for drinks containing sucrose or HFCS results in less weight gain, because these drinks provide fewer calories and most do not activate the survival switch. Our research group has also confirmed that sucralose and saccharin do not cause weight gain in laboratory animals. These studies suggest artificial sweeteners may be helpful for a person wanting to lose weight.

The problem, however, is that artificial sugars do not block the craving for sweets, and they might even encourage it. For example, a recent analysis of the National Health and Nutritional Exam Survey found that children who drank diet drinks consumed more caloric sugars on average than children who primarily drank water. This likely explains why some studies have found that people who drink diet soft drinks are at greater risk for gaining weight.

If you have a strong desire for something sweet, your best option is a whole fruit, not artificial sweeteners. Fruits can appease some of our hunger and craving for sugar, likely due to the effects of some of the flavonoids present.

> **Takeaway:** Use artificial sugars with caution, if at all. They do not cause weight gain on their own, but they also do not block craving for sugar and may encourage it. (Oh, such sweet sorrow.)

QUESTION 5.
I UNDERSTAND SOFT DRINKS ARE BAD, BUT WHAT ABOUT SPORTS DRINKS?

Should athletes use them, and can they also cause obesity?

Competitive sports and vigorous recreational activity are demanding. During strenuous exercise, we sweat to dissipate the heat that builds up in our bodies, but in so doing we lose water and salt. As a consequence, we can become dehydrated. Even mild dehydration (a loss of 2 percent of body water) has been shown to affect our ability to concentrate and perform.

The first sports drink was developed by Robert Cade, a physician at the University of Florida, in the mid 1960s. Cade became aware that the members of the university football team were becoming dehydrated in the Florida heat, and some of the players were losing more than ten pounds of weight during games. Although they were drinking water and taking salt tablets, it was not enough to prevent dehydration. Cade had attended a lecture at a national scientific conference in which he learned that the absorption of salt in the gut was markedly enhanced if paired with glucose in the rehydration fluid. Furthermore, when we exercise, we burn glucose (in the form of glycogen) in the muscle and liver, and Cade realized that providing some glucose could replenish this fuel for the muscles while protecting the athlete from developing low blood glucose. This led Cade and his team to create the first sports drink that contained water, salt, and glucose. The drink initially did not taste too good, as glucose is not that sweet. However, over time, the drink was improved by adding flavors and small amounts of fructose, and modern-day Gatorade was born.*

Many studies were performed around this time to identify the optimal content of sports drinks to improve performance. One of the first findings was that optimal performance occurred at a glucose concentration of 6 percent; higher concentrations actually hindered performance. Next was the discovery that the addition of small amounts of fructose to the glucose improved performance further, as the fructose enhanced the absorption of glucose in the gut and led to greater glucose delivery to the muscle and improved performance—even when total calorie intake was kept the same. Additional studies showed that the fructose content always had to be lower than the glucose content, for higher amounts of fructose caused a dramatic worsening in performance.

While there is debate, my ideal sports drink would be about 4 percent glucose and 1–2 percent fructose, with a salt concentration of about one-half gram per liter. This would provide about 4 or 5 grams of fructose in an 8-ounce

---

* Cade was a creative genius and very humble and funny. I had the pleasure of being his close friend and also the Robert Cade Professor at the University of Florida. One story he shared with me was from early in Gatorade's development. One of the first football players to drink his sports drink stated it tasted "like piss" and poured it over his head during a game instead of drinking it. Cade simply smiled and said that he may still have benefited from the drink because it helped him cool off.

drink—an amount small enough that it would be metabolized in the intestine rather than activating the survival switch.

By contrast, soft drinks, which are dehydrating and worsen performance, are about 6 percent fructose and 5 percent glucose. Similarly, when our collaborators administered solutions containing 5 percent fructose and 3 percent glucose to laboratory rats that were mildly dehydrated from heat stress, such solutions worsened their hydration status and caused kidney damage.

Takeaway: Sports drinks can prevent and treat dehydration during vigorous exercise, and also may help individuals suffering from illness who are dehydrated from diarrhea or vomiting. Having some glucose and small amounts of fructose leads to improved performance and does not increase the risk for obesity. I do not, however, recommend sports drinks when one is not exercising or ill.

QUESTION 6.
THERE ARE SOME REPORTS THAT SUGAR CAN IMPROVE PERFORMANCE. HOW IS THAT POSSIBLE, GIVEN THE EVIDENCE THAT SUGAR IMPAIRS SCHOOL PERFORMANCE?

You may have heard that, according to some studies, sugar can help improve mental performance, especially during intense exercise or when provided to children who skip breakfast. This is sometimes used as an argument to encourage sugar intake.

However, the "sugar" in these studies was not table sugar (sucrose) or fructose-containing sugars such as HFCS, but rather glucose. Also, many of these studies have been in children, in whom skipping breakfast has been shown to worsen school performance. Providing glucose can prevent this effect; too much glucose, however, may actually worsen performance. Consistent with these findings, a randomized study showed that adolescents receiving a low-glycemic breakfast performed better on standard tests assessing working memory and attention than children receiving a high-glycemic breakfast or no breakfast at all. Interestingly, glucose levels peaked around 115 mg/dL in the children who ate a low-glycemic breakfast, compared to 125 mg/dL among those who ate a high-glycemic breakfast.

Similar studies have been performed in adults, including university students and the elderly. They showed that memory is improved in fasting individuals given glucose, as is reaction time. Again, this appears to depend on the dose of glucose, as there is evidence that high doses do not offer any benefit.

> **Takeaway:** Low blood sugar worsens mental performance, but so does high blood sugar. Be sure to eat breakfast, but steer clear of cereals with high-glycemic indexes!

QUESTION 7.
ARE SOME PEOPLE RESISTANT TO THE EFFECTS OF FRUCTOSE-CONTAINING SUGARS? WHAT ARE THE POTENTIAL CAUSES OF SUGAR RESISTANCE?

There are some people who appear "resistant" to sugar, for any of several reasons. Young people, for example, seem able to eat sugar with impunity. But as we've seen, one explanation for this is more limited previous exposure to fructose. In individuals of any age who do not eat a lot of fructose-containing sugars, the systems for absorbing and metabolizing fructose are not "turned on." As a result, when they do eat sugar, they have a relatively mild metabolic response.

Another common reason is that young and/or athletic individuals tend to have healthier mitochondria. Their healthier energy factories are more resistant to the fructose-driven oxidative stress that triggers the survival switch. I would view neither of these situations as true sugar resistance, however, for if the individuals continue to ingest fructose-containing sugars, then the consequences of the fat switch will surface.*

Another group that is thought to be resistant to fructose is the Hazda, a group of modern hunter-gatherers living in Tanzania. The Hazda live on wild plants, figs, honey, and both small and large game. Honey is a major part of their diet, especially for the men; it can account for one-sixth of the calories they eat (and sometimes more). As you'd expect from such a high fructose intake, the Hazda suffer from substantial dental cavities and periodontal disease. Yet they remain lean and relatively free of diabetes and heart disease.

It is my opinion that the Hazda are not resistant to sugar at all. Rather, fructose from the honey they eat is what lets them make enough fat to survive. Game is not so easy to find for the Hazda, and the men spend much of the day walking long distances (around ten miles) to find food. Notably, despite exercising so much, studies show that they both eat and burn the same number of calories in the day as a sedentary office worker in New York. However, this is exactly what you would expect to happen with activation of the survival switch. While they may spend a lot of energy foraging for food, their bodies likely reduce how much energy they spend when at rest, so that the food they eat can help them survive longer. I believe the Hazda are eating just enough honey to help them survive. Without it, they would risk starving.

In contrast to the Hazda, the Guna people of the San Blas Islands off the north coast of Panama may have found a way to be truly resistant to sugar. Early reports dating to the 1940s suggesting that the people living on these islands were protected from developing high blood pressure led scientists to wonder if they might carry a protective gene.

Norman Hollenberg, a leader in cardiovascular medicine from the Brigham and Women's Hospital in Boston, went to Panama in the 1990s to investigate, and discovered that the Guna seem to be resistant not only to high blood pressure, but also to obesity and diabetes. However, he found that Guna who

---

* The fact that young people, and especially athletic individuals with healthy mitochondria, are relatively resistant to the effects of fructose is why you see such variability in studies where fructose is given to individuals. The HFCS industry prefers to give fructose to the young, athletic, and healthy, who will show only minimal metabolic effects from a single dose or short course of fructose—whereas the same amount of fructose given to an individual with obesity or insulin resistance results in a substantial metabolic impact.

had moved to Panama City were developing obesity and diabetes at high rates, suggesting that the protection was not due to genetics, but rather to something special about the way people lived on the islands. When he and his team looked at diet, they found that the Guna on San Blas were eating a lot of salt (roughly 12 g/day) and a lot of sucrose (table sugar). However, the group's dietician noted that they were also drinking lots of bitter cocoa every day—five to ten cups. Hollenberg, and then others, found that the cocoa contained a special type of flavonoid called **epicatechin** that appears to stimulate mitochondria growth, increasing the number of energy factories in the body and optimizing energy protection.

Our group investigated this further with the help of scientists Guillermo Ceballos, Francisco Villarreal, George Schreiner, and Sundeep Dugar. Volunteers with metabolic syndrome and high blood triglyceride levels were randomly assigned to take either an epicatechin supplement or a placebo for four weeks. At the end of that time, we observed improvement in blood triglycerides and inflammation markers with epicatechin, and also improvement in fasting glucose levels in those individuals who had been insulin resistant. We also showed that epicatechin could block the effects of fructose on liver cells by protecting the energy factories from oxidative stress. In short, epicatechin provides some protection against the development of metabolic syndrome. (We will talk about this more in chapter ten.)

Finally, there is another rare type of true sugar resistance that is observed in only 1 in 100,000 people or less: a genetic condition known as "**essential fructosuria.**" People with this condition do not have the ability to make fructokinase, the enzyme that breaks down fructose, and as such the survival switch cannot turn on. People with this condition live a normal life but can eat sugar without complication, as much of the fructose they consume is excreted in the urine. To date, no person with essential fructosuria has ever been reported to develop obesity or type 2 diabetes.

Takeaway: Sugar resistance is rare but exists. Most people who think they are resistant to sugar are not and will develop metabolic syndrome if they continue to ingest fructose-containing sugar over time. There are ways to become more sugar-resistant, such as eating and drinking less fructose, maintaining healthy energy factories by exercise, and possibly eating or drinking foods rich in certain flavonoids.

QUESTION 8.
IS THERE A WAY TO BLOCK OUR CRAVING FOR SUGAR?

The craving for sugar is a main reason people fail to reduce their intake. Is there anything we can do to block it?

While we cannot currently block craving outright, there are things we can do to reduce it. One of the best approaches is to go on a low-carb diet or simply dramatically reduce your intake of added sugars. This is associated with an initial intense period of severe craving that can last for several days, but the craving tends to decrease after the first or second week.

Note that reducing added sugars by replacing them with artificial sugars may, as mentioned, continue to promote sugar craving. Therefore, to successfully reduce sugar craving, you may need to eliminate artificial sugars from your diet. Similarly, because drinking alcohol is very much linked with the desire for sugar, it will help to reduce alcohol intake as well.

You could also attempt to appease your sugar craving with whole fruit. Some evidence suggests whole fruit may satisfy severe craving while not worsening metabolic syndrome.

Other methods of reducing craving include simulating fullness by drinking a lot of water or eating vegetables or salad; and distracting yourself, such as by exercising or visiting friends. Some investigators have also tried using various nutritional supplements, such as glutamine, but I am not aware of any strong evidence that these supplements are effective.

There may be a way to block craving just on the horizon, however. We know that animals that lack the ability to metabolize fructose do not seem to crave fructose and also do not develop metabolic syndrome when they eat it.

This has led to an effort by the pharmaceutical industry to make drugs that inhibit fructose metabolism. A benefit of such inhibitors is that they would also block the effects of the fructose we make from eating high-glycemic and salty foods. Today, several large companies are trying to make drugs that can block the effects of fructose, which could block craving as well. Our group is developing a drug that targets fructokinase, aimed at blocking the craving for both fructose-containing sugars and alcohol (the latter of which, as we learned in the last chapter, also goes through the fructose pathway).

> **Takeaway:** There is not yet a reliable way for us to block the craving for sugar. For now, our best option is to try all of the tricks we can to dampen our craving. My recommendation is to resort to a whole fruit when the urge for sugar calls you.

We may not be able to fully block craving (for now), but please do not despair, for the knowledge of the survival switch still allows us to develop a way to beat obesity. In the next chapter we will explore ways to turn down the switch, to prevent further weight gain and health problems, while in the last chapter we will use what we know to develop ways to lose weight, keep it off, and improve our health, too.

CHAPTER 9

The Optimal Diet for Blocking the Fat Switch

T o help protect animals at risk of death from starvation, dehydration, suffocation, and other threats to survival, nature developed a biological response (sort of like a 911 call) that we have named the survival switch. The primary way this switch is activated is by eating or making fructose; dehydration and elevations in blood glucose both "turn on" the body's ability to make fructose. Ingesting foods that are rich in umami can also activate this biologic switch, as these foods stimulate the production of uric acid, which has a critical role in fructose's effects. The importance of this pathway for survival is why we, and many other species, have developed specific tastes for sweet, salty, and savory foods.

The effects of the switch are quite powerful. First, it stimulates craving and impulsivity while reducing willpower, which helps drive foraging for food and water even in dangerous situations. It causes leptin resistance in the brain, so that we remain hungry even after we eat and therefore take in more food than we need, which allows us to build up our fat stores. It helps us conserve energy by decreasing our energy demands while we rest, allowing us to retain the fat stores we already have even as we spend energy foraging. There are also biologic changes going on unrelated to storing and burning calories, including development of insulin resistance (to reserve glucose for the brain), increase in blood pressure (to preserve circulation), stimulation of inflammation (to help protect us against infection), and oxidative stress in the mitochondria that slows energy production.

The consequence of this complicated process is that the calories we eat are redirected from immediate energy production to the production of fat, while we burn less fat. We compensate for the subsequent reduction in available energy by eating more (to help replenish our energy) and by shifting energy production to a primitive system that does not use oxygen.

This is an ideal system for protecting animals, us included, in the wild, but it was meant to be engaged for only limited periods. Today, we are chronically stimulating this pathway, and this carries adverse consequences that are driving obesity and many of our current diseases (metabolic syndrome, diabetes, high blood pressure, and others). To protect ourselves now, we must stop activating this survival switch–turned–fat switch. And that is the task we turn to here.

First, we must remind ourselves that the process we are discussing is not a simple on/off switch, but rather should be viewed as a dimmer switch, because the degree of activation can vary with the amount of fructose we ingest or make, and the speed with which we ingest or make it. In addition, an individual's response to turning up their switch will depend on their health. A healthy athlete with excellent energy factories will be less susceptible to the effects of fructose compared to a person who is already overweight and prediabetic. Likewise, older people, especially with other underlying conditions, are at more risk than the young.

I also want to acknowledge that there are certainly other factors that contribute to obesity besides the fat switch. These include the role of socioeconomics, education, cultural mores, genetics, the "enclosure effect" (see box on next page), and even the bacteria that live in our gut (the microbiome). Nevertheless, based on the studies I have performed and reviewed, I believe the fat switch is likely the major factor driving obesity, metabolic syndrome, and the diseases that result.

How, then, do we minimize activation of the survival switch? What diet should we eat—that can be maintained with relative ease—to prevent weight gain and maximize our long-term health?

THE ENCLOSURE EFFECT

One of the most overlooked reasons we gain weight is something I call the "the enclosure effect." Animals kept in a confined space where food is readily available often become fat. This is why there is an epidemic of obesity in the zoos, and why some pets become obese as well. Unlike the survival switch, which is a biological pathway driving food intake through hunger, the enclosure effect encourages eating as a habit, in response to boredom from being in a confined space. (Of course, if you then eat foods that activate the survival switch, you will add a biological desire to eat.) Many of us live in our own "enclosures," and this may play a role in our food intake.

THE BIG THREE

Let's start by looking at the three major nutrients: carbohydrates, fat, and protein. It is possible to have a healthy diet that does not require severe restriction of any of these, and that is our goal here. But when it comes to their activation of the survival switch, not all carbs, fats, and proteins are the same.

Good Carbs and Bad Carbs

The Western diet currently consists of 45 to 65 percent carbohydrates. Fifteen to 20 percent is added sugars, and the rest is complex carbohydrates, which include starchy and nonstarchy vegetables, grains, and nuts. Generally speaking, most books promoting a healthy diet have incriminated carbohydrates as the principal dietary factor driving our obesity epidemic, and as such many diets involve some type of restriction of carbohydrates, especially sugary and starchy foods, with a corresponding increase in protein and/or fat intake.

Our studies confirm these findings, but also incriminate other noncarbohydrate foods in activating the switch. Importantly, not all carbohydrates are bad. The ones we should be concerned with are the fructose-containing sugars, such as sucrose and HFCS, and carbohydrates that cause a significant rise in blood glucose levels. I believe other carbohydrates are not only safe to eat, but also beneficial to health.

A food's glycemic index, discussed in chapter five, can help us distinguish between carbohydrates that result in a strong elevation of blood glucose levels and those that do not. Some high-glycemic carbs include rice, potatoes, bread, cereals, and chips; low-glycemic carbs include most nonstarchy vegetables (such as broccoli and asparagus), salad vegetables (such as lettuce, cucumbers, and tomatoes), beans and legumes (such as lentils), and seeds and nuts. There is one other factor to consider, however, and that is whether a food has a high **glycemic load**.* This takes into account not only how likely the food is to raise your blood glucose (that is, its glycemic index), but also how much carbohydrate a normal portion of the food contains. Watermelon, for example, has a high glycemic index, but one slice will not raise your glucose too high, because there are not many carbohydrates in that single slice; it has only a moderate glycemic load. Spaghetti, on the other hand, has only a modest glycemic index, but because people often eat a lot at one sitting, it can easily raise glucose levels high enough to activate the survival switch.

Not all carbohydrates are bad.

Some of the more common high-glycemic foods and their glycemic loads are listed in the table on the next page. Foods with a high glycemic index (defined as >70) or with a high glycemic load (defined as >20) should be restricted in your diet. More complete lists of the glycemic index and glycemic loads are available online.†

---

* The glycemic load is calculated by multiplying the grams of carbohydrate present in a normal serving by the glycemic index, expressed as a percent. A glycemic load of 20 or more is considered high, and would be equivalent to eating 20 grams of white bread. For example, spaghetti has a low glycemic index (42), but the amount eaten in a serving is high (48 grams), so its load is high as well ($48 \times 0.42 = 20$).

† One site that lists the glycemic index and load of common foods is at https://www.health.harvard.edu/diseases-and-conditions/glycemic-index-and-glycemic-load-for-100-foods. A more complete list is provided in "International Tables of Glycemic Index and Glycemic Load Values: 2008," by Fiona S. Atkinson, Kaye Foster-Powell, and Jennie C. Brand-Miller, in the December 2008 issue of *Diabetes Care*.

Examples of Carbohydrates with High-Glycemic Index or Load			
Carbohydrate	Serving Size	Glycemic Index	Glycemic Load
Baked potato	1 medium	100	33
Instant oatmeal	1 cup	83	30
Cornflakes	1 cup	80	23
Watermelon	1 cup	76	8
White rice	1 cup	73	35
White bread	2 slices	71	20
Pancake	1 pancake	70	39
Bagel	1 bagel	69	24
Sweet corn	1 corn	60	20
Spaghetti	1 cup	48	20

When choosing between carbohydrates, there are some interesting additional things to consider. For example, instant oatmeal or instant rice, which only has to be heated briefly before being eaten, generally has a higher glycemic index than its noninstant counterpart. This is because the grain, so that it can be cooked quickly, has been preprocessed, which destroys or removes the fiber. There are also different types of starch. Starches are composed of stacks of glucose molecules that are broken down in the gut; one main type (amylopectin) is broken down much more easily than the other main type (amylose), and so has a higher glycemic index. Most white rice contains mainly amylopectin and is high glycemic, but long-grain rice (such as basmati rice) has a higher amylose content and so tends to have a lower glycemic index.

Also worth noting is that there is a lot of variation in how well individuals break down carbohydrates. One reason is genetics. For example, recall that some people can break down the amylose in starch much easier than others because they produce high levels of the enzyme amylase (see chapter five). The type of bacteria you carry in your gut can also change the way you break down carbohydrates. This has led some nutrition advocates to recommend the use of a continuous glucose monitor in order to determine your own personal blood glucose response to different types of food.

In contrast to high-glycemic carbohydrates, most vegetables are low glycemic and should be healthy, especially green vegetables. They do contain some fructose but at low amounts that appear insufficient to activate the survival switch, and multiple studies show they reduce the risk for obesity and heart disease.

MONITORING YOUR PERSONAL
BLOOD GLUCOSE RESPONSE

Because of the remarkable variation in blood glucose levels be-tween individuals in response to carbohydrates, you may wish to consider obtaining a continuous glucose monitoring device to pro-vide a personalized assessment. This device attaches to the back of the upper arm and provides minute-to-minute information on your blood glucose levels as you go about your day.

I personally have found this device to be useful in identifying what specific foods raise my blood glucose levels (and therefore have the potential to activate the switch) and also for identifying when I am susceptible to low blood glucose levels (<60 mg/dL), which can lead to light-headedness and confusion (the latter of which can occur during exercise, fasting, or restricting carbohy-drate intake).

A good goal is to maintain glucose levels between 70 and 110 mg/dL for most of the day. Glucose levels are expected to rise fol-lowing a meal, but the level of glucose one to two hours after eat-ing should be less than 140 mg/dL and ideally less than 120 mg/dL. While we do not know the specific glucose level in the liver or blood that triggers the survival switch, maintaining blood glucose levels in this range will certainly minimize the production of fruc-tose in response to carbohydrate intake.

Good Fats and Bad Fats

Before we talk about the different types of fat, it is important to discuss fat in general, and how it relates to the switch.

Fat was originally the main suspect in the mystery of what was causing the obesity and cardiovascular epidemics, as it is the most energy-dense food. A spoonful of fat has more than twice the calories as a spoonful of sugar; 9 calories per gram as opposed to carbohydrate's and protein's 4 calories per gram.

However, eating fatty food by itself does not activate the switch or, on its own, make you gain weight. Indeed, our collaborator, physiologist Phil Scarpace, performed studies in which laboratory animals were fed lard without any added sugars, and these animals did not become fat, as they remained leptin sensitive and adjusted their calorie intake as needed. Nevertheless, if the switch is already activated due to fructose-containing sugars or salty foods, then the addition of fatty foods leads to rapid weight gain because of their high caloric content. We showed this with Phil by first feeding fructose to animals to make them leptin resistant, then stopping the fructose and placing the animals on a lard diet. Because they were leptin resistant, they could not control their appetite, ate much more of the lard than normal laboratory rats did, and rapidly gained fat.

In other words, once we have lit the fire (that is, turned on the switch), fat makes that fire burn larger and brighter. This is why a diet that is high in both sugar and fat is the best way to make a laboratory animal obese. This is also of relevance to us, as the standard Western diet typically is high in added sugars and fat as well.

On a low-carbohydrate diet (and therefore a diet that is low in fructose and high-glycemic carbohydrates), the survival switch is turned down, and you are less hungry. Therefore, even though your diet may be high in fat, you will not gain weight. This is also why a low-fat diet only results in weight loss if you also include calorie restriction as part of the diet, whereas on a low-carb diet, calorie restriction (i.e., avoiding fat) is not required. Fructose is the criminal. Fat is only an accomplice.

Fructose is the criminal. Fat is only an accomplice.

There are several different types of fat. **Saturated fat** is the main fat in butter, coconut oil, palm oil, whole milk, cheese, fried foods, and red meats. While saturated fats do not have any known interaction with the survival switch, they have been implicated in raising LDL cholesterol (the bad cholesterol), which has been shown to be a risk factor for coronary artery disease. Accordingly, I concur with most medical societies in recommending saturated fats be limited to no more than 10 percent of daily calories.

Trans fats are fats made from a chemical process called hydrogenation, which changes vegetable oils from a liquid to a solid form to extend shelf life.

These used to be found in vegetable shortening, margarine, and a large number of packaged foods. Once considered safe, they were later found to increase the risk for diabetes and heart disease, and were banned by the FDA (although, as of this writing, trans fats can still be used to fry foods in some restaurants). There are small amounts of natural trans fats in some foods, especially beef, lamb, and dairy products, but some studies have suggested that these low levels of trans fats do not pose a threat. I am unaware of any way in which trans fats interact with the survival switch, but thankfully the question is moot in the United States now that trans fats have been banned from the market.

There are also monounsaturated fats and polyunsaturated fats. **Monounsaturated fats** are found in olive oil, canola oil, and peanut oil, as well as in avocados and sunflower seeds. Olive oil is the favorite one in the Mediterranean region, and has been associated with reduced risk for heart disease.* **Polyunsaturated fats** include both omega-3 and omega-6 fatty acids. **Omega-3** is primarily found in fish, especially oily fish such as salmon, mackerel, and tuna, as well as in walnuts, flaxseed, and unhydrogenated soybean oil. In contrast, **omega-6** is primarily found in corn oil, safflower oil, and all types of soybean oil.

Omega-3 fatty acids block many of fructose's effects.

Omega-3 fatty acids stand out as a very healthy fat that can block many of fructose's effects. Numerous studies suggest omega-3 fatty acids are beneficial for health, with salutary effects on blood triglycerides, blood pressure, heart disease, and kidney disease. Omega-3 fatty acids also appear to block some of the negative effects fructose has on cognition, at least in animal studies. Hummingbirds have high levels of omega-3 fatty acids in their muscles, which might protect their mitochondria from oxidative stress that would otherwise result from the high amount of sucrose-rich nectar they drink each day. In addition to being good for our brains and energy factories, omega-3 fatty acids also have important anti-inflammatory properties.

* Although both canola oil and olive oil contain primarily monounsaturated fats, olive oil is preferred, as canola oil can become oxidized more easily with heat, making it lose some of its health-promoting effects. Additionally, the ultrarefined nature of most canola oil may cause loss of protective micronutrients and polyphenols, and greatly diminishes its antioxidant content.

In contrast, studies on omega-6 fatty acids are variable. Some studies have found evidence that omega-6 fatty acids stimulate inflammation, leading some health experts to argue that the key to managing inflammation is to increase the ratio of omega-3 to omega-6 fatty acids in the diet. However, other studies have suggested that omega-6 fatty acids may be beneficial. Given that the literature on omega-6 fatty acids is mixed, my recommendation is to not focus on the amount of omega-6 we consume, but rather emphasize consuming foods high in omega-3 fatty acids.

Good Proteins and Bad Proteins

Protein normally accounts for 15 to 20 percent of our daily calories and is important not only for helping build muscle, but also for making different proteins that help us run the biologic processes we use to live. Increasing the amount of protein in the diet can also help people lose weight, as protein appears to be uniquely capable of quelling hunger, compared to fats and carbohydrates. However, there is some controversy as to whether this is due to a special ability of protein to stimulate satiety or to the fact that increasing protein intake generally results in a simultaneous reduction of carbohydrates.

While protein intake is important for many critical functions, there are good proteins and bad proteins. Most studies suggest that red meats (like beef, pork, and lamb) are distinctly harmful. They have been associated with increased risk for obesity, diabetes, heart disease, kidney disease, and cancer, links not generally observed for other types of protein, including other animal proteins (like poultry and most fish), dairy proteins, and vegetable proteins.

One reason red meats may be different is that they tend to be rich in inosine monophosphate (IMP), one of the umami substances that can be converted to uric acid to activate the survival switch. Shellfish, and some fish such as tuna, also contain a lot of IMP. In contrast, poultry and vegetable proteins tend to be lower in these substances. Not surprisingly, red meat intake is associated with the development of gout, while intake of poultry, dairy, and vegetable proteins are not.

Red meats tend to be rich in an umami substance that can activate the survival switch.

Ingestion of red meats can also lead to the generation of toxic substances. One such substance, **TMAO** (trimethylamine N-oxide), is a risk factor for heart disease. While its function in humans is unknown, it plays a survival role in fish, protecting their tissues from the effects of water pressure at ocean depths. So it is possible that it might also be linked with the survival switch.

Given these issues, I recommend poultry, dairy, and vegetable proteins over red meats. I also prefer fish to red meat, for while fish can be rich in umami, they also tend to be high in omega-3 fatty acids. Examples of plants that are rich in proteins include artichokes, asparagus, beans of all kinds (including tofu, which is fermented bean curd), cole crops (broccoli, cauliflower, brussels sprouts, cabbage, bok choy, collards, and broccoli), lentils and all dried and fresh peas, mushrooms, nuts and seeds, peanuts, oatmeal, potatoes, quinoa, spinach, and grains such as millet, quinoa, and wild rice.

COMPARING SUCCESSFUL DIETS

Given what we now know about the three major nutrients, I think it is useful to review some of the more popular and successful diets currently being used and evaluate their benefits and shortcomings when it comes to the survival switch. Then we can use this information to develop the ideal diet for blocking the switch's activation and therefore preventing weight gain and the development of metabolic syndrome.

One note before we start: The ideal diet is one that does not enforce calorie restriction, but rather naturally reduces caloric intake by quelling hunger—as occurs when blocking the survival switch (since one of the key consequences of the switch is inducing hunger through craving and leptin resistance). This is not to say that diets that force calorie restriction do not work for weight loss, for when your diet involves calorie restriction, you'll lose weight whether you are eating cardboard or steak.* The problem is that such diets do not address the underlying problem driving weight gain.

So let's compare some of the more popular diets for their ability to block the survival switch. I will not discuss conventional low-calorie, low-fat diets, as

---

* Most changes in weight are due to changes in calorie intake, but over time changes in metabolism are also important. How to improve your metabolism is discussed in the next chapter.

these tend to include high-glycemic carbohydrates and fructose-containing sugars that activate the switch and are miserable at preventing features associated with metabolic syndrome (likely a reason they do not reduce heart disease, even though they lower bad LDL cholesterol). Cross the traditional low-fat diet off your list.

Low-Carb and Keto Diets

The goal of low-carb diets is to reduce total carbohydrate intake. They include diets with only modest restriction (where carbs make up only 30 to 45 percent of calories in the diet, or 130 to 180 grams daily), classical low-carb diets (20 to 30 percent carbs, or about 80 to 130 grams daily), and ketogenic, or "keto" diets (5 to 10 percent carbs, or 25 to 50 grams daily). The most extreme keto diets usually require a dramatic increase in fat intake (65 to 70 percent) to make up for the reduction in carbohydrates, as it is very difficult to increase protein intake above 20 or 25 percent of calories.

Low-carb diets focus on reducing fructose-containing sugars and high-glycemic carbohydrates, which are two of the main triggers of the survival switch. They do not require caloric restriction because appetite naturally decreases, and they improve all features of metabolic syndrome. They can also be magnificent diets for people with diabetes, and in some cases are associated with the reversal of type 2 diabetes.

While I am a big fan of the classic low-carb diet, there are some drawbacks. For one thing, low-carb diets can be hard to maintain. While some have successfully remained on low-carb diets for years, attrition is high.

Low-carb diets also tend to increase LDL cholesterol (the bad cholesterol), and there have been rare occasions where cholesterol levels of individuals on these diets have reached 600 mg/dL or more.* However, for many individuals the change in LDL cholesterol is modest, and LDL particle size also tends to be larger and therefore less likely to cause heart disease.

My greatest concern is with ketogenic diets (as opposed to classic low-carb diets) and whether they are a good diet choice long term. Normally our bodies

---

* In the late 1920s, the arctic explorer Vilhjalmur Stefansson and his friend went on a diet of 1 percent carbohydrate, 20 percent protein, and 80 percent fat for one year, and their blood became milky with cholesterol of 800 mg/dL or higher. While they thought they were mimicking the Inuit diet, the percentage of fat in the Inuit diet is only around 50 percent.

maintain a certain level of glucose in our blood to provide enough fuel for the body, especially the brain and muscle. To help us maintain that blood glucose level, we store glucose as glycogen in our livers and muscles and release it as necessary between meals, and also make some glucose as needed from proteins and fat. When a person is on a severe low-carb diet, they use up most of their glycogen stores. They can still maintain their blood glucose levels from the protein and fat they eat, but glucose is generally less available.

Glucose is the brain's preferred fuel, so when less glucose is available, it should be dangerous for the brain. However, the brain can use another fuel: ketones, which are produced when the body burns fat. Ketogenic diets cause a glucose-deprived state that leads to the burning of fat and, with it, high levels of ketones in the blood, a state called ketosis. That's where the diet gets its name.

There is some evidence that ketogenic diets are well tolerated, and ketogenic diets have long been used as a treatment for epilepsy. Nevertheless, the long-term effects of ketosis are not well understood. Also, ketosis does affect exercise performance, as glucose and muscle glycogen are especially critical for high-intensity sports.

The amount of uric acid in the blood also increases during ketosis. We had previously shown that one effect of uric acid is to stimulate glucose production, and hence this increase might represent a compensatory mechanism to help maintain blood glucose levels. As such, I do not recommend lowering uric acid levels when on a ketogenic diet unless they are causing gout. Uric acid may have other effects, however, such as stimulating behaviors associated with the foraging response, which may not be ideal for prolonged periods.

In addition, the diet's reduction in whole fruit and vegetable intake may also not be beneficial long term. Indeed, studies have found that individuals whose intake of carbohydrates is chronically lower than 40 percent may suffer increased risk of mortality. However, good studies on individuals on true low-carb (less than 30 percent carbs) or ketogenic (less than 10 percent carbs) diets have not been done.

The Paleolithic Diet (A Type of High-Protein Diet)

The Paleolithic or Paleo diet is based on the diet of hunter-gatherers. Around 1.8 million years ago, during a period of cooling temperatures, *Homo erectus* first appeared. Consistent with his name, *H. erectus* stood upright. He also carried tools, hunted, and discovered fire—which could be used not only to protect against predators, but also to cook food, making meats and plants easier to digest. Our diet transitioned away from being largely plant based, heavy on fruit, seeds, and nuts, as the introduction of cooking increased meat intake significantly. This brought more of both protein and fat into our diet, and was associated with a drop in the energy needed for digestion, which reduced the size of the gut. In turn, there was more energy available for the brain, and brain size increased.

The Paleo diet emphasizes lean meats (such as wild game), fish, shellfish, and eggs. While leafy vegetables, fruits, berries, and nuts are not restricted, sugar, breads (including whole grains), potatoes, legumes (such as peas, beans, and lentils), dairy products, alcohol, and coffee are not allowed. This results in a diet high in protein (about 30 percent of calories) and fat (about 40 percent of calories), with modestly reduced carbohydrate intake (about 30 percent of calories).

Like the low-carb diet, this diet has many advantages. The high protein content coupled with the removal of high-glycemic carbohydrates and sugar results in a natural reduction in food intake, such that caloric restriction is not necessary. Features of metabolic syndrome substantially improve. One problem, however, is the high protein intake, which makes it a difficult (as well as expensive) diet to maintain. As we discussed earlier, high intake of red meats as well as umami foods such as shellfish can increase uric acid levels and raise the risk for diabetes and heart disease. The restriction of dairy products also eliminates the benefits of milk proteins and makes it more difficult to get enough calcium and vitamin D (see discussion later in this chapter). High-protein diets are a bad idea for people with chronic kidney disease, as there is evidence that they tend to worsen the disease over time.

The Mediterranean Diet (A Type of Plant-Enriched Diet)

The Mediterranean diet emphasizes vegetables, fruits, nuts, legumes, and whole grains. The diet also encourages the use of olive oil (a monounsaturated fat) in many dishes, and includes fish and seafood (which are rich in omega-3 fatty acids) at least twice a week. Poultry, eggs, and dairy foods are eaten in moderation, while red meats are eaten infrequently. Compared to the classic Western diet, it tends to include higher protein intake (20 percent of calories) and fat intake (35 percent of calories), and lower carbohydrate intake (45 percent of calories).

A 2020 study compared the Mediterranean diet with the Paleo diet and intermittent fasting in overweight adults when it came to weight loss, metabolic outcomes, and adherence over twelve months. The primary differences between the Paleo and Mediterranean diets were the Paleo diet's higher protein and especially red meat intake, and the Mediterranean diet's higher intake of whole grain and dairy products. Intermittent fasting involved severe restriction of food two days a week (to approximately 500 calories a day) with no restrictions in food content or intake the rest of the week.

All three diets appeared beneficial at six months for weight loss and improvement of metabolic parameters, including percent body fat, waist circumference, blood pressure, insulin resistance, and systemic inflammation. At one year, the weight loss was greatest in the intermittent fasting group, followed by the Mediterranean diet, while the metabolic parameters tended to improve the most in the group on the Mediterranean diet (especially insulin resistance and systolic blood pressure).

It's worth noting, however, that by the end of the first year, only about half of the individuals on the Mediterranean and intermittent fasting diets were still following the diet, and even fewer were still following the Paleo diet: only one-third. While all three diets appeared to provide benefits, this study favored the Mediterranean diet, as well as intermittent fasting, over the Paleo diet, possibly in part due to greater difficulty participants had staying on the Paleo diet.

INTRODUCING THE SWITCH DIET

Given the difficulty of maintaining existing diets, as well as the risks many of them carry, there is room for a new diet that may be easier to follow and should, thanks to our knowledge of the survival switch, lead to even healthier outcomes. Again, our goal here is a diet that will turn down the switch so we can prevent weight gain and maintain or improve metabolic health, not necessarily lose existing weight. (The next chapter will focus on how to use the switch to lose weight, and how intermittent fasting can be incorporated into this diet.)

Allow me to introduce the Switch Diet.

Compared to the standard Western diet, the Switch Diet involves a slight reduction in carbohydrates (about 45 percent of calories), with a slight increase in protein (20 percent of calories) and fat (35 percent of calories). It is similar to most people's current diet and hence may be easier to accommodate long term.

In terms of carbohydrates, the *initial goal* would be to reduce added sugars from the current intake of 15 to 20 percent of the diet to 10 percent (about 200 calories, 50 grams, or 12 teaspoons, based on a 2,000 calorie diet), consistent with the FDA's nutritional guidelines. The initially modest nature of this reduction will, I believe, make the diet more achievable. Nevertheless, no drinks with added sugars are allowed. The *long-term goal,* which hopefully would be achieved within a year, is to reduce added sugars to approximately 5 percent of intake, which is what the World Health Organization recommends.

For intake of natural sugars present in food, I recommend three or four servings of whole fruit each day, ideally separated. Fruits containing more than 8 grams of fructose per serving should be limited, or eaten in half-serving quantities. Dried fruits and fruit juices should only be eaten sparingly, if at all. Jams, jellies, applesauce, and other foods with concentrated fruits should generally be avoided, but you can review the amount of total sugars* per serving on these products' nutrition labels. If a serving contains fewer than 8 grams of total sugar, it represents 4 grams of fructose or less and is fine to eat. Sugar-free jams and jellies are permitted.

I recommend reducing high-glycemic carbohydrates, including rice, bread, potatoes, refined cereals, and large portions of pasta. Having a continuous glucose monitor can be helpful in determining how you individually respond to these foods; your goal is to keep your blood glucose level less than 120 mg/dL after a meal. In contrast, low-glycemic carbohydrates—especially vegetables and high-fiber foods—are generally recommended. One to two slices of whole grain breads and steel cut oats with minimal added sugars can be eaten daily.†

---

* When looking at a nutrition food label, look at *added sugars* as the sugars that count, EXCEPT for foods high in natural sugar, like fruit sauces, fruit juice, and honey, where you should look at the *total sugar* content.

† Whole grains tend to have a high glutamine-to-glutamate ratio and may help counter the effects of glutamate-rich umami foods. Recent studies suggest that individuals who have higher circulating glutamine levels compared to glutamate levels tend to have reduced cardiovascular mortality, and people who eat a diet with a higher glutamine-to-glutamate ratio also suffer less heart disease. While whole grains have high ratios, red meats tend to have low ratios.

COMMON DIETS

| Diet (Carbs/Protein/Fat) | FOODS THAT SHOULD BE RESTRICTED TO OPTIMIZE HEALTH | | |
	Added Sugars and High-Glycemic Carbs	Saturated Fats	Red Meat and Umami Foods
Western (55/15/30)	High	High	High
Low-Fat and Low-Calorie (60/15/25)	High	Low	High
Low-Carb (30/20/50)	Low	Moderate	Moderate
Ketogenic (10/20/70)	Low	High	High
Paleolithic (30/30/40)	Low	Low	High
Mediterranean (45/20/35)	Low	Low	Low

Omega-3 Rich Foods	Benefits	Risks
Low	None	Obesity Metabolic syndrome Heart diease Kidney disease
Low	↓ Weight ↓ Cholesterol	↑ Metabolic syndrome No benefit on heart disease
Moderate	↓ Weight ↓ Blood Pressure ↓ Metabolic Syndrome	↑ Uric acid ↓ Ability for high-intensity exercise
Moderate	↓ Weight ↓ Blood Pressure ↓ Metabolic Syndrome	↑ LDL cholesterol ↑ Uric acid ↓ Ability for high-intensity exercise
Moderate	↓ Weight ↓ Blood Pressure ↓ Metabolic Syndrome	↑ Uric acid
High	↓ Weight ↓ Blood Pressure ↓ Metabolic Syndrome	None

For proteins, I would group red meat and shellfish such as shrimp and lobster together and limit these foods to twice a week or less, while emphasizing a high-protein diet rich in fish, dairy, poultry, and vegetable proteins.

When it comes to fats, I would give preference to foods rich in monounsaturated fats (especially olive oil) or omega-3 fatty acids. Salad dressings that contain olive oil or walnut oil, for example, are superior to dressings that contain blue cheese. Saturated fats should be limited to no more than 10 percent of overall caloric intake.

Please note, however: you should always check with your doctor before beginning any new diet.

Quite coincidentally, our Switch Diet is consistent with dietary recommendations made by Dariush Mozaffarian of Tufts University to optimize metabolic and cardiovascular health. He developed his diet recommendations from evidence-based clinical medicine and trials, whereas our work stemmed from studies to understand the survival switch—yet, excitingly, the two different approaches developed similar conclusions, which further supports this dietary approach.

So far we've outlined guidelines around macronutrients. However, our research into the survival switch suggests recommendations in several additional areas.

Water and Salt

Obesity, as you'll recall, is a dehydrated state, but that observation, as well as the importance of hydration as means for preventing and treating obesity, is commonly unappreciated by nutritionists and dieticians. People with obesity show signs of dehydration, and many drink less than one-half liter of water a day. Therefore, remaining hydrated is a crucial component of the Switch Diet.

The easiest way to check if you are drinking enough water is to look at the color of your urine: dark yellow suggests you are not drinking enough. Normal urine output is about 1.5 liters a day, and an excellent goal is to drink enough water to reach 2.5 to 3 liters per day, which tends to produce urine with only a faint yellow color. Your doctor has more sophisticated ways to help determine if you are dehydrated. You can measure the salt concentration in your blood* or

---

* The blood salt test is known as serum sodium (Na).

how concentrated your urine is.* You can also have the copeptin in your blood measured, to assess your vasopressin level.

The European Food and Safety Authority recommends 2.5 liters of water intake a day for men and 2.0 liters for women.† Since much of the water we ingest is through our food, I recommend six to eight glasses of water a day for the average person. One approach is to drink a full glass of water at each meal and drink a glass or two between meals. In other words, whenever you eat or snack, get a glass of water to go with it. If you are in an environment that is either hot or arid, you may need to drink more.

Salt intake should also be restricted, because salt, like drinking sugary beverages, can also cause dehydration. Most people eat 10 to 12 grams of salt daily, but the Institute of Medicine's recommended amount, and mine, is around 5 to 6 grams.‡ Major sources of salt are processed foods, some packaged foods, canned soups, and fast foods. For example, a fast-food cheeseburger and fries can contain as much as 3 grams of salt, while a homemade cheeseburger and fries may contain less than half a gram. Likewise, a ready-made, take-home package of risotto from the grocery store can contain over 3 grams of salt, while homemade risotto may contain less than a quarter of a gram. Beware as well of the common practice of injecting meats, fish, and shrimp with salt and water to make them look bigger. I discovered this once when the shrimp I was grilling shriveled up to half their size as the water came out (leaving the salt behind).

Other heavily salted foods include french fries, chips, and popcorn. When I would eat popcorn at the movies (a ritual in my family), I always noted that my weight would go up the next day. I had assumed this was water weight from holding on to the salt, but our work suggests that some of the weight gain might have been from the acute effects of salt on increasing glycogen in the liver.

---

* Dehydration is indicated by a high urine osmolality (>500 mOsm/kg) or high urine specific gravity (>1.020).

† The recommendations for children are, unsurprisingly, somewhat lower: 1.6 L daily for children four to eight, and 1.9 L/d and 2.1 L/d for those age nine to thirteen, respectively. Children over age fourteen receive the same recommendation as adults.

‡ Salt (or sodium chloride) contains about 40 percent sodium. Sometimes you will see recommendations for sodium intake instead of salt intake. In this case, 1 gram of salt is about the same as 400 mg sodium.

If you must eat salty foods, drink a lot of water. Drinking water before you eat salty food may even prevent the development of thirst and the activation of the switch. Or try to replace salt with some other seasoning, such as coriander, dill, garlic, ginger, lemon juice, onion, paprika, rosemary, sage, tarragon, or vinegar, that provides flavor without activating the switch.

Finally, it is possible to drink too much water. People can become water intoxicated, a state in which salt concentrations in the blood fall significantly (a condition called hyponatremia) and cause headache, continuous yawning, and nausea. In rare cases, it can progress to life-threatening conditions such as seizures and coma. The risk for water intoxication is increased during marathon running or other intensive exercise, as well as following surgery, especially gynecologic surgery.* Some health conditions, such as heart failure or kidney disease, may also increase the risk for water intoxication. To avoid this condition, aim for eight 8-ounce glasses of water per day as a general rule. If you are in a marathon or engaging in intensive exercise, drink only until your thirst resolves. Finally, if you have any significant health condition, ask your doctor what they recommend.

Umami Foods

Our research led to the discovery that umami foods (foods containing glutamate or the nucleotides AMP and IMP) activate the survival switch by directly stimulating the production of uric acid.† This observation was disappointing for me, as savory umami foods have often been considered safe and even healthy.

However, in our experiments, you had to give a laboratory rat a fair amount of these substances to trigger weight gain. Therefore, I believe that small amounts of umami foods are likely okay, such as anchovies with a salad, a few oysters, a dab of blue cheese dressing, or some dried tomatoes.

One major exception is beer. I do recommend reducing or eliminating beer (a hard task for many, I know; see page 188). I also recommend limiting dishes extremely rich in umami such as sardines and shellfish (for example, shrimp,

---

* The reason gynecologic surgery is associated with increased risk of water intoxication is not known, but young women undergoing surgery are particularly susceptible.

† Patients with gout are frequently told to eat foods low in **purine** content, as purines are converted in the body to uric acid. In fact, most purine-rich foods are also rich in umami, as AMP and IMP are broken down to purines in the process of making uric acid.

crab, and lobster). Furthermore, if you have high blood uric acid levels (>6 mg/dL in women or >7 mg/dL in men), you may want to be even more stringent when it comes to umami foods.

Umami-Rich Foods					
Drinks	Meats	Seafood	Cheese	Vegetables	Condiments, Sauces, and Extracts
Beer	Organ meats	Oysters, clams, mussels	Blue cheese	Dried tomatoes	Soy sauce
Tomato juice	Red meats	Shrimp, crab, lobster	Roquefort	Seaweed (kombu)	Fish sauce
	Duck	Squid	Gorgonzola	Mushroom (shiitake)	Gravy and meat extracts
		Anchovies, sardines	Parmesan	Spinach	Yeast extracts
		Dried bonito flakes (tuna)		Broccoli	Kimchi
		Mackerel		Soybean	
Italicized foods have greater glutamine, AMP, and/or IMP contents and carry higher risk.					

Dairy Products

Milk proteins appear to counter the survival switch by reducing uric acid levels, which are associated with lower risk for both gout and diabetes, so dairy products are generally recommended. Unsweetened dairy foods are also associated with less risk of obesity, diabetes, and heart disease. The standard fortification of milk with vitamin D also confers benefits, especially as uric acid has been shown to interfere with vitamin D metabolism.

Since the saturated fat present in whole milk and cheese may increase risk for higher cholesterol levels, reduced-fat dairy products such as low-fat milk or yogurt may be superior. However, whole milk and butter are likely fine if your LDL cholesterol levels are within a healthy range (<100 mg/dL*). Most cheese is also fine, although cheeses that are high in umami should be limited, such

---

* This target level is for the average person. It is a good idea to consult with your physician, as sometimes a lower LDL cholesterol is recommended depending on your overall health.

as those with high yeast content (that is, blue cheese, gorgonzola, Roquefort) and aged cheeses such as Parmesan. Ice cream is fine if it is low in carbohydrates (such as low-carb ice cream to which maltitol has been added as a sweetener). However, it may encourage craving for sweets, and hence I recommend it be reserved for special occasions.

Coffee, Tea, and Chocolate

Coffee directly counters the survival switch, as one of its metabolites can block the formation of uric acid. This is likely why one study reported that drinking five cups of coffee a day (without added sugar) is associated with a 50 percent lower risk of developing diabetes or gout. While caffeine is a stimulant, it does not have significant effects on blood pressure. Given these findings, I encourage coffee, although five cups a day is too much for me!

Teas—especially green teas, and again without sugar—are also generally healthy. Many contain flavonoids, those substances present in plants that have multiple (generally healthy) biological effects. Some flavonoids, for example, have been shown to block the survival switch as well, although weakly. (We'll discuss the use of flavonoids in the treatment of metabolic syndrome in the next chapter.)

Cocoa, at least from grocery stores, tends to include sugar and is not recommended, although a bitter cocoa drink like the one the Guna drink may aid in blocking the switch. Dark chocolate (chocolate with 70 percent or higher cocoa content) is recommended. One ounce (30 grams) provides between 30 mg and 40 mg of epicatechin, which is the active ingredient in chocolate that has protective effects against metabolic syndrome. An alternative would be to take epicatechin daily as a supplement (doses range from 30 mg to 300 mg), although the purity and potency of these supplements appear to vary.

Alcohol

Alcohol should be considered a type of sugar, as, like glucose, it can trigger the activation of the polyol pathway and result in the generation of fructose. Hence, alcohol directly activates the switch. All drinks are not equal, of course. Beer is especially bad, as the brewer's yeast present in it is, as we've discussed, an umami food that also activates the switch. Many drinks involve mixing alcohol with juices or soft drinks. Rum and sweet wines such as sherry and port also have a high sucrose content.

For many of us, alcohol may be hard to quit—even harder than sugar. For beer lovers, I recommend first reducing beer intake to one small serving of beer at a sitting, and then gradually replacing that beer with unsweetened wine. I would suggest the same for those who like hard alcohol. Whatever alcohol you drink, be sure to sip rather than drink it fast, and drink water between sips. This will help keep the concentration of alcohol in your blood low so that the generation of fructose is minimized.

One glass of wine with a meal can be enjoyable and is associated with good health, in part because of favorable effects on cholesterol (especially good HDL cholesterol). Two glasses are acceptable on occasion. However, the take-home message is that alcohol acts like sugar, and should be treated accordingly.

Vitamin C

Finally, I recommend supplemental vitamin C, which helps block the switch, both by stimulating the excretion of uric acid in the urine and blocking the effects of uric acid on the body's energy factories. Limit the dose to 500 mg to 1,000 mg daily, as higher doses can be associated with an increased risk of kidney stones—another reason to stay well hydrated, as hydration reduces this risk.

The Switch Diet	
Sugar	• Reduce sugar intake to 10 percent of daily calories (with 5 percent as a long-term goal). • Eliminate sugary drinks entirely.
Carbohydrates	• Reduce high-glycemic carbohydrates. • Emphasize whole grains, low-glycemic vegetables, and high-fiber foods. • Limit fruit to 3–4 servings daily, separated, with half servings for high-glycemic varieties. • Avoid dried fruit, fruit juices, fruit syrups, and fruit concentrates.
Protein	• Limit high-umami proteins (red meats, organ meats, and shellfish). • Emphasize fish, poultry, dairy, and vegetable proteins.
Fat	• Emphasize monounsaturated and omega-3 fats. • Saturated fats can account for up to 10 percent of total caloric intake.
Salt	• Reduce salt intake to 5–6 grams daily. • Limit processed foods, as they are often high in salt (as well as sugar).

Water	• Drink 8 ounces of water 6–8 times a day.
Dairy	• Dairy is generally recommended, especially milk. • Butter and cheese are fine if LDL cholesterol levels are controlled. • High-umami cheese should be limited.
Coffee, Tea, and Chocolate	• Coffee and tea are recommended. • Dark chocolate is encouraged.
Alcohol	• Reduce or eliminate alcohol. • If you must drink, sip rather than drinking quickly, and alternate with water.
Vitamin C	• Take a vitamin C supplement daily.

LOWERING YOUR URIC ACID

Uric acid, you may recall, is generated during fructose metabolism and has a significant role in driving metabolic syndrome. High levels in the blood (>6 mg/dL in women and >7 mg/dL in men) are strongly associated with obesity, diabetes, and high blood pressure. As such, I recommend you have your blood uric acid levels measured, for they will tell you whether you are at increased risk for developing these conditions.

If your uric acid level is high, changing your diet should be your first approach to reducing it. This includes reducing intake of all foods that can activate the switch, but especially sugary beverages and foods, and also umami-rich foods that can produce uric acid directly. However, some people will continue to have elevated uric acid levels in the blood even after changing their diet. In such cases, should you consider taking a medication to lower your levels?

If you have a history of gout, you should for sure take a medication such as allopurinol, with the goal of lowering your uric acid level to 6 mg/dL or below (for both men and women). As we saw in chapter six, there is increasing evidence that uric acid can crystallize not just in the joints, but multiple sites throughout the body, including the coronary arteries, aorta, and kidneys. Since gout is evidence of uric acid crystals in the joints, bringing uric acid levels into the normal range minimizes the risk of crystals forming and causing damage in other locations.

By contrast, the idea of receiving treatment for high uric acid levels with no history of gout is controversial. Many small clinical trials suggest that lowering serum uric acid is of benefit: that it has the potential to lower blood pressure in people with hypertension, improve insulin resistance, reduce systemic inflammation, help reduce fatty liver, improve kidney function, reduce weight gain, and sometimes even drive weight loss. However, not all trials showed positive effects. In most cases this is likely due to faulty study design, such as evaluating the effects of lowering uric acid on people with already normal levels, or on the blood pressure of healthy subjects without hypertension (both situations in which no benefit would have been predicted). Nevertheless, more clinical trials are needed to resolve the controversy. Treatment of elevated uric acid levels in the absence of gout is currently not approved by the FDA.

The diet we've outlined here is aimed at preventing weight gain and improving overall health. And while this dietary advice may incidentally lead to weight loss, it is not specifically aimed at helping you lose weight. Let's turn to that next.

CHAPTER 10

Restoring Your Original Weight and Improving Your Healthspan

Mark Twain once said that quitting smoking was easy, as he had done it thousands of times. One could say the same thing about losing weight. It is relatively easy to lose weight, and many of us can count numerous times when we went on a diet and succeeded in losing enough pounds that it was noticeable to our family and friends. The literature is full of diets that have claimed success in achieving weight loss. However, losing weight is not where the problem is. Rather, it is the regaining of weight. For many, these diets are hard to maintain, and eventually our old habits return. Our weight slowly increases to where it was when we started, only to stay that way until we once again make another attempt to diet.

This also carries implications for our health. While it is true that there are individuals who are overweight or with obesity who appear to be otherwise healthy, we know from studies that these individuals are still at increased risk for developing diabetes and high blood pressure, as well as other conditions. Being overweight for long periods of time may limit our **healthspan**, the period of time in our life when our overall health is good and we have the energy to enjoy life, making the ability to not only lose excess weight but keep it off incredibly important.

Dieticians and nutritionists have tried to prevent the regaining of weight through intensive counseling, use of social groups in person and online, telephone reminders, podcasts, and/or apps that can help you count, record, and report the calories you are ingesting, with the hope that these things will keep you on track. Others actually design your meals. Some diets place you on calorie restriction, and suggest ways to divert your hunger when it occurs. Yet, despite all of these measures, it is not only hard to get to the weight you want, it is even harder to maintain that weight for any substantial period.

For those who do manage to get back to their ideal weight and stay there, some are lucky enough to return to the energy and lifestyle they remember. However, for others, maintaining their diet and exercise plans continues to require constant vigilance and immense emotional and mental drive.

We discussed earlier how dieticians and nutritionists originally viewed the failure to maintain weight loss as a consequence of the challenges of living in Western society, where the need for exercise is minimal while access to fast food, junk food, and processed food is easy. However, scientists and biologists are now painfully aware that the inability to maintain weight loss is not simply due to Western society and culture. An inability to restore our weight and health is not a consequence of poor decision-making or deficient moral strength. Just as there is a biology to explain why we gain weight, there is also a biology to explain why it is difficult to maintain weight loss. Most importantly, our research into the survival switch can explain this biology, and, even better, provide the needed solutions.

> *An inability to restore our weight and health is not a consequence of poor decision-making or deficient moral strength. It's biology.*

WHY DO SO MANY PEOPLE REGAIN WEIGHT AFTER SUCCESSFUL DIETING?

Numerous studies have been performed in an attempt to understand the biology of why people regain weight after successful dieting. The complete answer so far remains both unknown and a hot area of nutrition research. Nevertheless, I believe that the knowledge we have obtained from understanding the survival switch can provide answers to this mystery that will allow us to develop ways to prevent weight regain. This means that one day we will not just treat obesity and the health risks that accompany it, but rather cure them.

The primary biological problem is that, when you have been overweight or obese for a while, your body begins to think of your current weight as normal. Indeed, it wants to keep you at that weight. This means that when you go on a diet and begin losing weight, your body responds by reducing how much energy it uses. This decrease in your metabolism minimizes your weight loss. You may also get hungrier, which drives you to eat more to regain the weight you have already lost.

This carries an unpleasant consequence for those who lose weight by dieting. Eating the same plate of food that kept you in balance before you started to lose weight now causes weight gain. You have to eat *less* than you used to or you will gain the weight back. And the more weight you lose, the less you can eat. This is likely why even the world record holders for fasting never got to their original weight. When you fast for an extended period, the energy you need decreases in response, sort of like it does for an animal that is hibernating. Since you are using less and less energy to function, weight loss slows down over time. For all of the good things associated with fasting, it is still not enough.

Most of us want to weigh the same as we did in our youth, but it is a tough life if we have to eat one-half of what the person next to us eats, despite being at the same weight. It is as if your body wants you to have that extra fat, while you want to have normal food intake and lots of energy. Yet now it seems as if this is impossible. I refer to this as being "locked in."

A POSSIBLE CAUSE OF GETTING LOCKED IN TO A HIGHER WEIGHT

Recall that most of the energy we make comes from our energy factories, or mitochondria. This energy is in the form of ATP, and it is used to drive our biological processes and maintain our body metabolism. When we eat fructose, it produces uric acid that causes oxidative stress to these energy factories. This in turn reduces production of ATP while shunting the calories from fructose into storage as fat and glycogen. The process allows us to build up stores of energy for times when food is not available.

As mentioned earlier, the oxidative stress that occurs as a consequence of activating the switch can be damaging, both to the energy factories and the rest of our body. However, in nature, this oxidative stress is typically short lived, and the energy factories recover. We, in contrast, are turning on the survival switch full blast for years and years. What was meant to be a temporary depression of energy production by the mitochondria for survival purposes becomes a permanent one, with dire consequences.

When exposed to chronic oxidative stress over time, structural changes occur in the energy factories. They become smaller, and mitochondrial function decreases. They produce less energy *even when the switch is not activated*. This resets the metabolism, lowering energy production and use as weight increases. Because your body now thinks the higher weight is its normal weight, it sees weight loss as a threat to your survival and responds by altering your metabolism further. At this point, your metabolism is your enemy!

The consequences of chronic switch activation are not simply about weight or even energy. There is even some evidence that chronic or recurrent oxidative stress drives the aging process—that it is responsible for wrinkles and the slow wear and tear on our internal organs. All food intake is associated with some oxidative stress to these energy factories (and, in fact, this is why reducing caloric intake may enhance life span, as discussed in chapter one). However, fructose intake causes much more oxidative stress to the mitochondria than other nutrients.

This suggests to me that curing obesity is easiest if it is caught early, before there is permanent damage to the mitochondria. Indeed, my personal experience has been that it is much easier to treat obesity in children and adolescents, and can be done simply by modifying diet to reduce intake of foods that can activate the switch. This is because younger people still have plenty of functioning mitochondria. In contrast, for people who have been obese for years, it can be very challenging to treat them, for their energy factories have been experiencing chronic oxidative stress for a long time. Yet, it can still be done. The key is rehabilitating the mitochondria.

THE WAY TO CURE OBESITY IS TO INCREASE ENERGY PRODUCTION IN YOUR MITOCHONDRIA

While the idea that we become locked in to higher weights and lower energy levels sounds very depressing, these conditions do not have to be permanent—it is possible to restore our energy factories. There are two major ways to approach this. First, we want to minimize damage to the energy factories so they have time to recover naturally. This approach focuses primarily on blocking continuous activation of the survival switch. Second, we want to proactively stimulate the repair of the energy factories, or, even better, increase the production of mitochondria to replace the ones we have lost.

Before we discuss how to do these two things, I want to provide a simple method whereby you can assess the health of your own energy factories: evaluating your natural gait, or the speed at which you normally walk. One way to do this

It is possible to restore our energy factories.

would be to record the time it takes to walk around the block while wearing a pedometer that counts your steps, then calculate both the number of steps and distance you walked per second. An easier approach is to simply record how much time it takes to walk around the block and compare that time with future walks to determine if your mitochondrial health is changing. The important part is that you want to be measuring your natural gait; in other words, you do not want to be purposely walking fast.* Normal gait speed is around four feet per second, but can range from two to six feet per second. I would set four or more feet per second as your goal. People who have been overweight a long time often have a lower gait speed, averaging around three feet per second.

Studies have shown that natural gait speed correlates with the quality of your mitochondria, and that individuals with a faster gait live longer and maintain better overall health. A reduced pace has been associated with increased fatigue and low ATP levels in skeletal muscle. Notably, people who are young and overweight tend to walk at a speed similar to other young people, but the

---

* This method is not useful if your ability to walk is limited by physical or neurological disabilities.

difference in gait speed between being overweight and normal weight becomes much more noticeable with age.

I encourage you to go for a walk and gauge your natural pace. Not only will this provide insight into how easy it will be for you to lose weight and keep it off, but monitoring your natural gait speed over time can be helpful in assessing overall progress.

BLOCKING THE FAT SWITCH

In the last chapter, we discussed ways to minimize activating the survival switch, including reducing intake of added sugars such as table sugar and HFCS, choosing low-glycemic carbohydrates over high-glycemic carbohydrates, and drinking plenty of water while reducing salt intake. How do these dietary changes affect our energy factories?

We were able to look at this in a clinical trial performed in Mexico City by researchers Magdalena Madero and Gaby Sánchez-Lozada, in which overweight individuals were placed on a modest low-salt diet (6 g of salt/day or less) or a low-salt and low-fructose diet (20 g of fructose/day). After eight weeks, there was a sixfold increase in mitochondria in the low-salt group's circulating white cells, and a *seventyfold* increase in white cell mitochondria in the low-salt, low-fructose group. (It would have been ideal to know whether the mitochondria were increasing in other important organs, like the brain, liver, and muscle, but that data was not available.) These results were encouraging: energy factories appear to improve when we reduce fructose and salt in the diet.

Another approach to reducing activation of the survival switch is **intermittent fasting**. This can be done in a variety of ways, including within the day (for example, a 16:8 plan, where sixteen hours of the day are spent fasting with an eight-hour period in which eating is allowed) or where fasting is done on various days of the week (for example, a 5:2 plan, where two days are spent fasting every week, while food intake is normal the other five days). There is a certain appeal to intermittent fasting, as it mimics life in the wild, and during the fasting period the switch is not activated. In addition to reducing overall calorie intake and being associated with weight loss, intermittent fasting appears to offer other benefits linked with reduced activation of the switch, such as a reduction in oxidative stress to the energy factories. Some studies suggest that it can even stimulate the growth of mitochondria. Intermittent fasting is also associated with a reduction in the risk for insulin resistance and diabetes, the development of systemic inflammation, and the development of Alzheimer's disease.

While blocking injury to the mitochondria is critical to preserving them, this alone is not enough to let us lose weight and keep it off, especially if we have been overweight for a long time. Beyond curbing intake of salt and fructose, how can we do this? A clue can be found by studying a special group of people that are, in essence, superhumans: elite athletes.

STIMULATING MITOCHONDRIAL GROWTH: LESSONS FROM SUPERHUMANS

I have a friend, Iñigo San Millán, who was a professional athlete for several years (competing in both soccer and road biking) before he became a physiologist who devotes much of his effort to understanding the exceptional performance of elite athletes. His work (as well as that of others) has demonstrated that top international athletes—which he has referred to as "superhumans"—have superb energy factories and, as a result, possess something he refers to as "metabolic flexibility," the ability to move back and forth between using fat and carbohydrates for energy. For example, when working out at low or moderate intensity, these athletes primarily burn fat, but when working out at full exertion, they primarily burn carbohydrates. In contrast, people with obesity are metabolically *in*flexible. As they cannot burn fat very well, they can only exercise for short periods of time, and their maximum oxygen consumption is only about one-third of the elite athlete's—suggesting that their energy factories, which require oxygen to function, are working less hard.

One of the most remarkable discoveries made by Iñigo is the importance of lactate in metabolic flexibility. Lactate, the circulating form of lactic acid, is what causes muscle fatigue. It is generated in muscle during the metabolism of glucose, and has historically been viewed as a dead-end waste product. However, it turns out that individuals with healthy mitochondria, like elite athletes, use the lactate as an additional energy source, taking it up into the energy factories where it is used to make more ATP. As such, they can exercise for a long time before lactate accumulates and they have to either stop exercising or significantly decrease the intensity. In contrast, people with obesity have trouble using lactate as an energy source, so it accumulates more rapidly, affecting both how long and how intensely they can exercise. Thus, how quickly lactate accumulates can provide an accurate measurement of how healthy an individual's mitochondria are, and of how metabolically flexible the individual is.

Iñigo has also shown that high lactate levels can impair mitochondrial function, similar to uric acid. It is therefore interesting that fructose generates much more lactate when it is metabolized than glucose, with nearly 25 percent of fructose eventually being converted to lactate. It suggests that another way fructose may negatively affect our energy factories is through its ability to stimulate lactate production.

Elite athletes' high energy production doesn't just allow them to break world records in international athletic competitions. It also protects them from developing obesity, diabetes, heart disease, and cancer. They do not need to be on any special diet, such as a low-carbohydrate or high-protein diet, to see these effects. In fact, they often prefer carbohydrates, as they are the most important energy source for muscles during high-intensity exercise and help keep glycogen levels in the muscle high.

Superhuman elite athletes have more productive energy factories than anyone else in the world. But why is that? Why are their energy factories so effective? While there are likely many factors, including genetics, one of the most exciting reasons is that exercise itself can stimulate mitochondrial growth. The trick, however, is that the exercise must be done a certain way.

INCREASING YOUR ENERGY FACTORIES

What is the best type of exercise to improve mitochondrial function? Many studies have examined this. First, it needs to be an endurance type of exercise, such as walking, exercising on a treadmill, swimming, or cycling, as opposed to a non-endurance activity like weight lifting.* Second, it is most effective if you are either fasting or do not eat any carbohydrates before the exercise. Third, the exercise has to be sustained for at least one hour, and be done at least three or four times a week. This is because it takes some time to activate the process of mitochondrial growth, and exercising less than thirty minutes at a time rarely achieves this.

Exercise intensity also matters. As Iñigo showed, once you start to accumulate lactate in your blood, not only do you begin feeling fatigued, but the high lactate levels block the mitochondria's ability to burn fat, resulting in an inability to continue exercising. So, the trick, for our purposes, is to find an exercise intensity where you can last an hour without accumulating lactate. This varies dramatically among individuals. People with poor mitochondrial function, like those with long-standing obesity or metabolic syndrome, have to exercise at a much lower speed than weekend or competitive athletes.

While the most accurate approach to determining the right exercise intensity is to buy your own lactate kit and measure your lactate level, there are also some tricks to achieving the exercise intensity you want. The simplest (and the one that Iñigo recommends) is considering the intensity of your breathing and your ability to talk. The right exercise intensity should allow you to maintain a conversation, but with some degree of difficulty. If you can speak and breathe while exercising almost as well as you can at rest, then you are going too easy. If you can't maintain a conversation, then you are exercising too hard.

Exercise is often categorized by zones based on heart rate. The level of exercise that is optimal for improving your mitochondria is referred to as Zone 2 exercise (Iñigo calls it "Z2"), and generally corresponds to light intensity characterized by a heart rate approximately 70 percent of your maximum healthy heart rate. Some individuals will use tables and formulas to calculate the heart rate they should target for Zone 2 exercise,† but unfortunately, these methods are poorly validated. There can be significant variation among individuals in maximum heart rate, meaning you may be targeting the wrong training zone to maximize your mitochondria. Also, medications such as beta blockers can

---

* Some studies suggest walking or exercising on a treadmill is superior to cycling. However, both methods are effective and you should choose whichever one you personally prefer.

† A common formula is to calculate your target heart rate for Zone 2 exercise by taking your maximum heart rate, estimated by subtracting your age from 220, then multiplying this by 0.7.

make reaching a calculated heart rate difficult. Therefore, I would favor having your lactate measured during exercise, or else following the simple talking test described by Iñigo. Either way, I recommend discussing with your physician what heart rate is safe for you prior to initiating this or any other exercise program.

The power of exercise is not simply in burning calories or making you stronger. Nor is it just in giving you a sense of satisfaction, achievement, or pleasure (that "runner's high" you may have heard about). The main benefit of exercise is to keep your energy factories strong and to stimulate their growth. This, in turn, helps prevent becoming locked in to a higher weight and unable to sustain weight loss after dieting. Indeed, my collaborator, national obesity expert Paul MacLean, showed that exercise helped prevent the regaining of fat in obese laboratory rats after they lost weight from dieting.

There are a few things other than exercise that can stimulate the production of energy factories lost from chronic activation of the survival switch. One is intermittent fasting, as discussed earlier. There is also some evidence that you can stimulate the growth of mitochondria with specific supplements (sometimes referred to as "exercise in a bottle").

One of the more potent ways of stimulating mitochondrial growth is by taking an epicatechin supplement. As you may recall, this is the substance present in dark chocolate and in the bitter cocoa that helped protect the Guna from obesity. It is also present in the seeds of the Brazilian guarana fruit. Aztec runners, famous for transmitting messages more than 250 miles in less than a day, were known for drinking large amounts of bitter cocoa, which may help explain their record distance runs. Green tea contains a similar but less potent substance known as epigallocatechin. Both dark chocolate (chocolate with 70 percent or higher bitter cocoa content) and green tea may therefore be beneficial for mitochondrial function.

Other supplements are often used to boost mitochondrial function, such as carnitine and co-enzyme Q, but whether these supplements can help increase mitochondrial number has not, to my knowledge, been determined.

You should also take care to avoid supplements that might impede your efforts to rehabilitate your energy factories. Supplemental antioxidants such as N-acetyl cysteine, alpha lipoxin, and vitamin C, while beneficial in blocking the oxidative stress that causes mitochondrial injury, ironically may also interfere with the rebuilding of mitochondria. So while I recommend vitamin C supplements for people who are at their desired weight and want to block activating the survival switch, I would not take this supplement in doses above 500 mg/day if you are trying to lose weight. Here the main goal is to increase your mitochondria, and some studies suggest that vitamin C doses of 1,000 mg/day may hinder that process despite having benefits for metabolic syndrome in general.

Overall, exercise remains the most established and proven way to improve your energy factories. My main recommendation is to walk fast, cycle, or run such that you pass the simple conversation test and to do this several times a week.

ANOTHER BENEFIT OF BETTER MITOCHONDRIAL FUNCTION: BLOCKING THE EFFECTS OF AGING

If we can protect and regrow our energy factories, we may also have an opportunity to slow the aging process and help maintain cardiovascular and brain health. Aging is thought to be due to the chronic effects of oxidative stress, especially to the mitochondria. This raises the possibility that chronic fructose ingestion might accelerate aging—and that stimulating mitochondrial growth could provide an antidote.

There are studies that suggest high sugar intake may shorten life span, in addition to increasing the risk of cardiovascular mortality and dementia. An example comes from studies of the fruit fly, scientists' favorite medical research subject. This little fly with its brick-red eyes loves to haunt kitchens and outdoor dining areas, searching for its favorite food: ripe fruits rich in fructose.

What happens when the fly is offered liquids containing sucrose? The fruit fly loves them! When the fly drinks the sugar water, it becomes fat and diabetic, just like us, and then dies young of dehydration and kidney disease, the cause of which appears to be related to uric acid. Highly concentrated sugar shortens the life of fruit flies even though they normally live on fructose from fruits.

Our group found provocative evidence suggesting that the chronic production of fructose in our body may contribute to aging as well. As we have learned, our bodies can make fructose from the glucose in carbohydrates, even if the carbohydrates do not contain fructose. To study this, we gave a high-carbohydrate diet containing less than 5 percent fructose to two groups of mice—one normal, and the other genetically modified so that they could not metabolize fructose—until they were old (approximately two years). The normal mice showed classic changes of aging, with mild aging-associated kidney damage and the rise in blood pressure we expect with age. The kidneys, vascular function, and blood pressure of the mice that could not metabolize fructose, however, remained normal.

What this suggests is that aging may be driven by low-grade activation of the switch over time. One would suspect that, if high intake of sugar had been included, the aging changes in the normal mice would have been further accelerated. Blocking the switch, coupled with improving our mitochondria, could add many additional healthy, high-quality years to our lives.

A PLAN TO LOSE WEIGHT AND KEEP IT OFF

In the previous chapter, we laid out a long-term diet, based on our knowledge of the survival switch, that can prevent us from gaining weight while maximizing our health and protecting us from diabetes, heart disease, dementia, and cancer. The goal in this chapter is different, for here we want to develop a diet to help those of us who are overweight lose that excess fat and keep it off, regain our youthful energy, and do so in a way that is safe and beneficial to our overall health. The key question is how knowledge of the survival switch can help us achieve this goal.

The first step of an effective weight-loss plan is to stimulate fat burning. Since we burn fat only when we need additional energy, we need to reduce the energy we obtain from our diet. All diets aimed at weight loss involve calorie restriction. However, the most successful diets *also* always involve turning down the switch, for this helps minimize hunger and the foraging response that occurs when the switch is turned on. This is why diets focused primarily on calorie restriction, but in which sugar and high-glycemic carbohydrates are allowed, are doomed to fail as soon as the calorie restriction ends. This is also why diets that *restrict* sugar and high-glycemic carbohydrates can cause weight loss even without specifically restricting calories. By dimming the switch, these diets reduce hunger, so caloric restriction occurs naturally. In addition, turning down the switch allows one to burn fat more effectively, for as you'll recall, one of the actions of the switch is to block the burning of fat (see chapter three).

The second step is to block the reduction in metabolism that the body uses to compensate for the weight loss and keep us at our current weight. As mentioned, when we have been overweight for a long time, our energy factories are working at reduced capacity, and this is associated with the body's perception of overweight as the new normal. When this happens, we respond to weight loss by reducing our metabolism, so that the amount of food that once kept us at a stable weight now causes weight gain. This process causes almost all dietary plans to fail. To overcome this, we have to prevent further injury to these energy factories by dimming the switch while we both stimulate the production of new energy factories and increase our energy output.

Currently the best approach to growing new energy factories is exercise—as we discussed, of a specific type. Importantly, the primary benefit of exercise is to stimulate our energy factories, not to burn calories. While the latter is beneficial, the best way to reduce available calories, in order to trigger the burning of fat, is diet. Indeed, if the switch is active, exercising to burn calories will be compensated by a further reduction in metabolism during rest. This is how animals that are starving compensate for the energy they lose when foraging for food. This is also why the Hazda can spend all day walking to find food without increasing their overall energy expenditure: activation of the survival switch through large amounts of honey means their bodies compensate for this exercise by reducing energy expenditure when at rest.

The primary approach I would recommend to achieve sustained weight loss is to begin with a low-carb or keto diet. The reason is that these diets heavily restrict added sugars, which are our main dietary sources of fructose, as well as the high-glycemic carbohydrates that are our main dietary sources of glucose, which the body can convert to fructose. By turning down the switch, these diets will reduce hunger naturally, and also allow the burning of fat, which the switch previously blocked. These diets also will "reboot" your

If the switch is active, exercising to lose calories will be compensated by a further reduction in metabolism, and doom our weight-loss goals.

system so that you no longer absorb and metabolize fructose as rapidly, as is the case when you are regularly eating a high-fructose diet (see chapter eight). This will make you more resistant to the effects of sugar on the limited occasions you do eat it.

These diets also reduce your glycogen stores. Recall that the body stores both fat and carbohydrates, the latter in the form of glycogen. When we fast, our body burns the glycogen first, since it prefers glucose as its fuel. If we are snacking on carbohydrates throughout the day, the fat stores in our belly are preserved. But by reducing our intake of carbohydrates, especially those that are either high glycemic or contain fructose, we minimize our glycogen stores and therefore increase fat burning. This is one reason why restricting carbs is so effective.

Our body's preference for glycogen as fuel also helps explain why sleeping eight hours or more is so helpful, and why exercising in the morning (prior to eating breakfast) is more effective at causing weight loss than exercising at night. When we sleep, we burn most of our glycogen stores, so that when we wake up, we are in fat-burning mode. When we exercise at night, we are primarily burning the glycogen we have accumulated over the day.

Finally, a low-carb diet may boost mitochondria growth, as suggested by our studies investigating low-fructose and low-salt diets.

There are some caveats with low-carb and keto diets. First, the risk of low blood sugar increases. If you feel sweaty or light-headed, you may want to check your blood glucose and/or eat a piece of fruit (despite it being a carbohydrate).

Second, some foods you can eat on a low-carb diet still activate the switch, such as salty foods and some umami-rich foods (for example, red meats and shellfish). Salty foods, as you recall, activate the switch by stimulating the conversion of glucose to fructose. However, when you are on a low-carb diet, there is relatively less dietary glucose available to be converted to fructose. As such, while you are on a low-carb diet, a high-salt diet is less likely to generate fructose, and thus less likely to cause weight gain. However, rich umami foods could still carry significant potential for weight gain. Also, consider reducing or eliminating alcohol intake, since alcohol can activate the switch as well.

A low-carb diet may also reduce blood pressure as a consequence of dimming the switch. If you are on blood pressure medication, you may want to follow your blood pressure carefully, as you may need to reduce your dosage.

Reducing salt intake and carbohydrates at the same time may also lead to low blood pressure, so if you become light-headed, you may want to check your blood pressure in addition to your blood glucose. Because of this, I recommend waiting until you have been on a low-carb diet for a few weeks before reducing your daily intake of salty foods, as well as other foods that can activate the switch.

Additionally, I recommend drinking at least eight glasses of water daily to ensure you remain hydrated, and monitoring both your bad LDL cholesterol levels and your blood uric acid levels. Occasionally, LDL cholesterol can rise significantly on a low-carb diet; if so, you will want to reduce the amount of saturated fat you are eating. Uric acid levels may also rise on a ketogenic diet, as mentioned in the last chapter. The biological consequence of the increase in uric acid, as noted previously, is unknown, but it may be a compensatory attempt to help maintain blood glucose levels (because uric acid stimulates insulin resistance) and blood pressure. However, it also causes oxidative stress to the energy factories. If your uric acid increases to very high levels (such as >8 mg/dL), you may want to weigh the risks of treatment against the potential benefits with your personal physician (see the previous chapter).

While some people can maintain a low-carb diet for years, for most people it can be difficult to stay on one for more than a few months. This is in part because of our natural desire for a greater balance of carbohydrates in our diet. Thus, I suggest an alternative dietary approach for weight loss.

If you would prefer not to go on a low-carbohydrate diet, you could instead use either a Mediterranean diet, or my Switch Diet, but be more stringent in restricting foods that can activate the switch. This means severely restricting intake of high-glycemic carbohydrates, particularly rice, potatoes, bread, chips, and cereals. If this, too, proves challenging, you could modify the diet whereby a small portion, perhaps half a serving, of a high-glycemic carbohydrate is allowed at just one meal a day, eaten slowly over an hour. At other meals, only low-glycemic carbohydrates would be allowed, with full restriction of other foods that can activate the switch, such as salty or umami-rich foods and alcohol. On some days, you could intermittently fast during the day using a 16:8 schedule to enhance calorie restriction, and stimulate growth of energy factories. (Importantly, there's some evidence that fasting can impair performance, especially in children—who I would not recommend use intermittent fasting regardless—so keep that in mind.) This latter plan results in slower weight loss, but may be more tolerable for many people.

Regardless of which method you choose, you'll want to exercise at least one hour, three to four days a week, focusing on staying in Zone 2. (Some groups, such as the World Health Organization, suggest that, in addition to light-intensity exercise, there may be additional benefits to including 75 to 150 minutes of high-intensity exercise a week. However, this is optional for our purposes, as it is Zone 2 exercise that will have the best effect on increasing your energy factories and let you burn the most fat.) Also, consider recording the distance and time of your walks to see if your natural gait is improving, which would suggest your energy factories are becoming healthier. Last, as suggested for the Switch Diet in the previous chapter, I recommend drinking plenty of water and eating an ounce of dark chocolate daily.

As a final point: I do not recommend *persistent* fasting for weight loss (although I recognize that this is what happens in nature, so it is possible I am wrong). While Angus Barbieri may have been able to fast a year, laboratory studies performed several months after he initiated his fasting showed his blood glucose levels were very low, around 30 mg/dL, occasionally dropping to 20 mg/dL. These levels of glucose are so low that, if they occurred suddenly in you or me, we would fall into a coma, with risk of permanent brain damage or death. The physicians treating Barbieri felt he was thinking fine, although they did not do any formal testing, and it is likely that his brain and other tissues were using the ketones generated from fat burning as the main source of energy, since there was minimal glucose around. But while studies show the brain can use ketones, my belief is that the body prefers glucose for a reason and I personally would want to keep my blood glucose levels in the normal range. More studies are needed to resolve this issue.

A Switch-Informed Dietary Plan to Lose Weight

To Stimulate Fat Burning	
Diet	• Low-carb or keto diet preferred, especially for the first month.
	• Switch Diet or Mediterranean diet (with more stringent restriction of high-glycemic carbs, salty foods, and umami) may be used as an alternative.
	• Drink at least eight glasses of water a day.
	• Reduce salt intake to 5–6 grams daily (though you may want to ingest more if you sweat a lot during exercise, and you can be more liberal with salt if you are on a low-carb diet).
	• Intermittently fast one or two days a week as tolerated, using a 16:8-hour schedule (optional).
	• Minimize or avoid alcohol.
Supplements	• Daily vitamin C supplement of 500 mg or less.
To Rebuild Your Energy Factories	
Exercise	• One hour, three to four times a week, in Zone 2.
Diet and supplements (optional)	• Dark chocolate or epicatechin.
	• Green tea.

A Few Final Words

When I started my research into obesity and metabolism, fructose was viewed simply as a component of sucrose and HFCS that gave sugar its sweetness. There was some evidence that sugar might be linked with obesity, insulin resistance, and high triglyceride levels, but many people thought these developed primarily due to excessive calorie intake, to which sugar was one of many contributors.

The last two decades have led to a whirlwind of remarkable research that has radically changed how we think about this simple sugar. What we have learned is that, for animals in nature, fructose is the grand savior, triggering an alarm that activates a wide variety of survival responses. The problem is that we now unnecessarily sound this alarm every day. Unlike with Chicken Little, however, the sky really is falling. Chronic, excessive activation of this survival switch is driving many of today's diseases. But as our understanding of this great disease process continues to increase, we can develop ways to overturn the powers of nature, and return to health and harmony.

In these pages I have presented research from my laboratory and those of my many collaborators on the discovery of that switch. This process followed the conceptual and innovative thinking of Steven Benner, an exceptional scientist whose quest is to understand the origin of life. Benner has suggested that, to best solve questions in science, one should study it using multiple disciplines and methods, an approach he refers to as "planetary biology."

A broader approach can provide solutions to a problem that might be missed by standard scientific investigation. Drilling down on a specific subject can offer incredible insights, but there is also much to be gained by "climbing a ladder" instead and getting a more general view on the subject. In our case, we embraced classic laboratory and clinical studies, but have also heavily favored understanding how nature views obesity as well as insights from evolution and history.

It is important to recognize that the survival switch is a hypothesis based on scientific studies. A hypothesis is a proposal, and experiments are designed to test that proposal. Experiments produce data, and if the data do not support the hypothesis, we adjust the hypothesis and repeat the process. My point is that new data from other scientists' studies (or our own) could contradict our survival switch hypothesis. If that occurs, we would then amend our hypothesis and continue the cycle. To date, I believe our proposal of the survival switch is the best hypothesis to explain the data available. Nevertheless, as scientists, we must keep open minds.

Our studies have some limitations. Much of our work is done with laboratory animals, especially studies showing that the body can make fructose. Laboratory animals are not human beings, and while we can extend our hypotheses from laboratory animals to humans, we cannot repeat many of our studies on humans, because we cannot genetically alter humans to knock out genes as we did with mice. Different studies have to be designed to test these hypotheses in humans. Nevertheless, studies have already confirmed that soft drinks do not just provide fructose from ingestion, but rather triple the *production* of fructose in humans, so data in human studies are coming. Likewise, we need more studies to help resolve some of the persistent controversies over the role of uric acid in metabolic disease.

The importance of the survival switch will ultimately be tested once clinically potent and safe inhibitors of fructose metabolism are on the market. Various pharmaceutical companies are developing drugs to block fructose metabolism. We have also identified some nutraceuticals that can block fructose metabolism, such as mangosteen and osthol, but more work is required to find out whether they are safe and effective in humans.

We still have a long way to go before obesity, metabolic syndrome, and type 2 diabetes become historical diseases, and there remains much science to be discovered. In this regard, I am reminded of a story commonly attributed to the philosopher Bertrand Russell, although it may not have originated with him. While traveling through India, Bertrand meets an old soothsayer who says she knows the secret of what holds up the world. Curious, he asks her if she could share it with him.

"Bertrand," the old woman says, "the answer is easy. The earth sits on the back of a large turtle."

Russell, thinking her logic is not strong, questions, "So if the turtle carries the earth on its back, what about the turtle? What is it standing on?"

"It's no use, Bertrand," the soothsayer replies with a smile. "It's turtles all the way down."

While this story is often used to exemplify the futility of looking for certain kinds of answers, it also depicts a common challenge in science: often, one must pass through many layers before reaching a root cause. It is much like a detective story, or an archaeological excavation, where one finds something of importance, and this leads to the discovery of another important insight, which leads to another insight, and so on, in a process that can seem endless.

You might say that, when it comes to the science of obesity, there remains a large bale of turtles left to be found. We need to generate new hypotheses and collect more evidence to solve the many mysteries that continue to challenge us. As Sherlock Holmes said, "Remember, once you eliminate the impossible, whatever remains, no matter how improbable, must be the truth."

Finally, I would like to leave you with a poem that came to me one day while I was out riding my bicycle through the park, and that sums up what I now know about sugar:

AN ODE TO SUGAR

From crushed cane comes a liquid sweet and clear,
Boiled and filtered until it is pure,
Yielding a virgin powder, soft and white,
With crystals like snowflakes, like stars in the night.

Sugar takes foods to heavenly heights,
Fluffy pies, chocolate cakes, and caramel delights.
Like fairies that dance with frosted wings,
Sugar brings pleasure, happiness, and dreams.

But woe to those who desire too much,
For they fall into trouble, as from Midas's touch.
What was driven by want is now forced by need.
What was given from love is now hoarded in greed.
What once satisfied the heart now takes from the soul;
What once brought love, now leaves the heart cold.

With fury the body fights this dark force,
Yet little can be done to stave off its cursed course.
The blood floods with sugar that rises to new heights,
The heart becomes swollen; the liver creamy white.
The teeth, once white, are rotten and stained,
The kidneys are dusky, shriveled, and inflamed.
Blood vessels are fatty, and may close off or burst,
Causing weakness, paralysis, dementia, or worse.
And Cupid's honeyed arrow that brought love and romance,
Now pierces the heart with a sugar-tipped lance.

Oh Sugar, my love, you must let me go,
And let me recover my heart and my soul.
The sweet pain you gave me can no longer stay;
Please give me the strength to turn you away.
The sweetness of your lips I will forever adore,
But to live my life, I need my health once more.

Acknowledgments

I thank my literary agent, Jennifer Herrera, and my editors, Leah Wilson, Nancy Hall, and Mary Ann Timeus; without their help, this book would not have materialized.

The research presented represents years of effort by many collaborators, for which I provide only a partial list. I especially thank Miguel A. Lanaspa, Gaby Sánchez-Lozada, Takahiko Nakagawa, Duk-Hee Kang, Yuri Sautin, Takuji Ishimoto, Bernardo Rodriguez-Iturbe, the late Jaime Herrera-Acosta, George Schreiner, and Marilda Mazzali, all of whom had large roles in many of the important discoveries. I also thank my research team, Ana Andres-Hernando, Wei Mu, Carlos Roncal-Jimenez, Christopher Rivard, David Orlicky, Gabriela Garcia, Olena Glushakova, Xiaosen Ouyang, Tamara Milagres, Katherine Gordon, Christina Cicerchi, Nanxing Li, and Zhilin Song. Thanks are owed as well to our visiting scientists and research fellows, including John Kanellis, Christine and Michael Gersch, Pietro Cirillo, Marcelo Heinig, David Long, Karen Price, Uday Khosla, the late Waichi Sato, Wei Chen, Fumihiko Sasai, Federica Piani, Yoshifura Tamura, Wataru Kitagawa, Katsuyuki Tanabe, Tomoki Kosugi, Mohamed Shafiu, Takahiro Nakayama, Thomas Jensen, Yuka Sato, and Masanari Kuwabara.

For clinical research studies, I thank Manal Abdelmalek, Reem Asad, A. Ahsan Ejaz, Petter Bjornstad, Claudio Borghi, Diana Jalal, Mehmet Kanbay, Ada Kumar, David Maahs, Magdalena Madero, Roberto Pontremoli, Janet Snell-Bergeon, Enrique Perez-Pozo, Jacek Manitius, Ebaa Al-Ozairi, Jillian Sullivan, Shikha Sundaram, Guillerom Ceballos, Myphuong Le, Xueqing Yu, and the late Chris King; and for basic research collaborations, I thank Paul MacLean, Mehdi Fini, Fernando Garcia-Arroyo, Joshua Rabinowtiz, David Bonthron, Leo Joostens, Thomas Finger, and Susan Kinammon. Thank you as well to my collaborators in New Zealand (including Tony Merriman, Gerhard Sundborn, and Simon Thornley) and Florida (Mark Segal, Phil Scarpace, Rajesh Mohandas, Bhagwan Das, and Sergei Zharikov). For the work on the chemistry of uric acid, I thank Alexander Angerhofer, Christine Gersch, Witcha Imaram, and the late George Henderson. For work on the development of fructose inhibitors, I especially thank Dean R. Tolan, Sundeep Dugar, Paul Maffuid, William Greenlee, Kai Hahn, Vijay Kumar, Soyoung Bae, Chase Needham, Michael Wempe, Tim Van Dyke, and my brother Todd Johnson. For work on alcohol dependence, I also thank Sondra Bland, Richard Bell, Esteban Loetz, and Richard Montoya.

I thank my friends with expertise in evolutionary biology and anthropology, especially Peter Andrews, Steven Benner, David Carn, John W. Fox, and Eric Gaucher, as well as my colleagues in the field of neurology and behavioral science, especially Fernando Gomez-Pinilla, my brother David Johnson, and William Wilson.

I also thank my collaborators studying nature and comparative physiology, including Peter Stenvinkel, Bruce Rideout, Johanna Painer, Paul Shiels, Lise Bankir, Barbara Natterson-Horowitz, Tanja Hess, Sandra Martin, and Greg Florant.

I also want to thank the Living Closer Foundation for their efforts to educate children on sugar and its role in obesity and diabetes. I give an especial thanks to Iñigo San Millán for allowing me to share his work on improving mitochondrial function by exercise.

Finally, I want to express my appreciation to Peter Attia, Michael Goran, Robert Lustig, Joseph Mercola, David Perlmutter, and Gary Taubes for their important books and podcasts, which have had a great impact on public education regarding the effects of sugar on health.

Glossary

Added sugars: Sugars that are added to foods, of which sucrose (table sugar) and high-fructose corn syrup (HFCS) are the most common.

Adenosine monophosphate (AMP): A nucleotide produced as a breakdown product of ATP. AMP is broken down to IMP and uric acid as part of the energy depletion pathway that turns on the survival switch. Like IMP, it is also a food additive that can enhance umami taste.

Adenosine triphosphate (ATP): The immediately available energy that we use to run our body.

Adipose: The medical term for body fat. Adipose collecting in the abdominal area is especially common in people with metabolic syndrome.

Allopurinol: A popular medication used to lower uric acid levels. Allopurinol is commonly given to people with gout.

Amylase: An enzyme that helps break down starch. It is produced by both the salivary glands and the pancreas. Salivary amylase levels tend to be higher in people living in agricultural communities than in other populations.

Attention deficit/hyperactivity disorder (ADHD): A behavioral disorder in which an individual, child, or adult manifests hyperactivity, inattention, and impulsiveness.

Bipolar disorder: A condition characterized by episodes of mania followed by episodes of depression.

Body mass index (BMI): A measurement, calculated from weight and height, that is often used to determine an individual's relative amount of obesity. A BMI of 20 to 25 is considered in the normal range, with overweight defined as a BMI of 25 to 30, and obesity as greater than 30. BMI may not reflect the true level of obesity in a muscular individual.

Calories: A unit of energy used to describe the amount of energy in food. One calorie is the amount of energy needed to raise the temperature of 1 gram of water by 1 degree Celsius.

Complex carbohydrates: Carbohydrates consisting of multiple sugars, connected in long, complex chains, that are broken down into glucose. An example is starch.

Diabetes, type 1: A condition in which blood glucose levels get extremely high due to the pancreas's inability to make insulin. The disease results from loss of the insulin-producing beta cells in the pancreas.

Diabetes, type 2: A condition in which blood glucose levels get extremely high, due initially to insulin resistance. Later there is also a loss of insulin production. Sugar intake is a major risk factor.

Dopamine: A substance produced in the brain that generates a pleasure response. Dopamine release is triggered by both caloric sugars and artificial sugars.

Energy depletion pathway: A series of chemical reactions that occur after fructose metabolism causes ATP levels in the cell to fall. The reaction begins with AMP being converted to IMP and eventually uric acid. It is sometimes referred to as the adenine nucleotide turnover pathway.

Epicatechin: A flavonoid found in dark chocolate that counters fructose effects by stimulating mitochondrial growth. Besides dark chocolate, it is also present in the guarana fruit. A related compound is epigallocatechin, which is in green tea.

Essential fructosuria: A rare disease in which the enzyme that breaks down fructose is absent. Individuals with essential fructosuria can eat fructose without risk of developing obesity or metabolic syndrome.

Estivation: A type of hibernation that occurs during hot temperatures (typically summers).

Fat switch: This is the same as the survival switch, except that the intake of fructose is so great that it drives obesity and diabetes, as well as a host of other conditions.

Flavonoids: Plant compounds that often have beneficial properties. Many are present in fruits and vegetables.

Foraging response: The behavioral response associated with animals seeking food. This includes the willingness to enter unfamiliar areas and take risks, and the ability to make rapid assessments.

Fructan: A chain of fructose molecules present in some plants. Humans cannot break down fructans. However, fructans can be converted to fructose by some gut bacteria, which makes them a stealth source of fructose; and by bacteria in our mouths, causing dental cavities.

Fructokinase: The first enzyme in the metabolism of fructose. This is the enzyme that triggers the initial depletion of ATP that stimulates the survival switch.

Fructose: The main sugar in fruit and honey. This is the sugar that triggers the survival switch.

Glucose: The primary sugar the body uses as fuel. Blood glucose is sometimes referred to as blood sugar. If blood glucose levels are too low (hypoglycemia), they can cause light-headedness and confusion; if too high (hyperglycemia), they can be a sign of insulin resistance or diabetes, especially if levels are chronically high. In food, glucose molecules are often bound together, forming starch in plants and glycogen in animals.

Glycemic index: A measure of how much a food raises blood glucose when compared to purified glucose. Pure glucose has a glycemic index of 100, while foods with a high-glycemic index have values of 70 or higher.

Glycemic load: Similar to the glycemic index, but taking into account the amount of food ingested. For example, spaghetti may have a moderate glycemic index, but large amounts of spaghetti tend to be eaten at one time, resulting in a more significant rise in blood glucose, and so it has a high glycemic load.

Glycogen: The principal way carbohydrates are stored in animals. It is similar to starch in plants.

Glycolysis: Whereas most of our energy is made in the energy factories (mitochondria) of our cells, some energy can be made through a primitive system called glycolysis. This system does not require oxygen to make ATP.

Gout: A type of arthritis commonly caused by the formation of uric acid crystals in the joints, typically that of the big toe. Gout is associated with obesity and metabolic syndrome and is precipitated by consuming sugar, umami foods, and alcohol (especially beer).

Healthspan: Similar to life span, but referring to those years in which one remains in good health.

Hibernation: A specific process in which animals store up fat and then go into a deep sleep during the winter. Hibernating animals have reduced metabolism.

High-fructose corn syrup (HFCS): A sweetener made from corn that contains a mixture of fructose and glucose. It has several advantages as a sweetener: its liquid state means it can be easily mixed into foods, it does not crystallize when frozen, and it tends to be inexpensive.

High-glycemic foods: Foods that can be broken down to glucose rapidly, and as such can lead to a rise in blood glucose after a meal. Typically these are foods rich in starch (potatoes, rice, crackers, bread) or sugar (sucrose or HFCS).

Hyperuricemia: Elevated serum uric acid, typically considered greater than 7 mg/dL in men and 6 mg/dL in women.

Inosine monophosphate (IMP): A nucleotide made from AMP that is part of the energy depletion pathway. Like AMP, it is also a food additive that can enhance umami taste.

Insulin: A hormone released by cells in the pancreas. Its primary action is to stimulate the uptake of glucose in muscle, liver, and fat.

Insulin resistance: A survival response in animals that acts to preferentially direct glucose to the brain as opposed to the muscle or liver.

Intermittent fasting: A dietary approach in which fasting and/or severe food restriction is done either within a given day (such as for sixteen hours of the day) or within a week (typically two days per week).

Ketones: Breakdown products generated during the burning of fat that can be used as fuel by the brain and other tissues when no glucose is available.

Knockout: A term often used to refer to an animal that does not have a particular gene, usually due to intentional removal through molecular biological techniques. A uricase knockout mouse, for example, lacks uricase.

Leptin: A hormone produced by the adipose tissue that gives us a sensation of fullness (also called satiety) that encourages us to stop eating.

Leptin resistance: Animals that have activated the survival switch are typically resistant to the effects of leptin, as are most people who are obese. Leptin is still produced, but the brain does not respond, and so hunger persists.

Low-grade inflammation: A condition in which our body's immune system is partially turned on despite no infection being present, measured by elevated markers such as C-reactive protein in the blood. Low-grade activation of the immune system likely helps protect animals from infection in the short term, but when persistently activated in people with obesity and metabolic syndrome, it increases the risk for kidney and heart disease.

Metabolic syndrome: The syndrome associated with storing fat. Typically, this includes elevations of triglycerides in the blood, increased abdominal girth, elevated blood pressure, and insulin resistance. Many individuals also have low HDL cholesterol (often referred to as the good cholesterol). Metabolic syndrome can be induced with fructose. Other names for this syndrome include *fat storage syndrome* and *syndrome X*.

Metabolic water: The burning of fat produces approximately 1 gram of water per gram of fat. This is called "metabolic" water.

Mitochondria: The specific components within the cell where ATP is produced in large quantities. Also referred to as the cell's energy factories. Mitochondria require oxygen to make ATP, distinguishing it from the primitive system known as glycolysis, which makes energy even when oxygen is absent.

Monosodium glutamate (MSG): An amino acid commonly added to food that activates the savory or umami taste (the fifth taste alongside sweet, salt, bitter, and sour).

Monounsaturated fat: A type of dietary fat found in vegetable oils such as olive oil, canola oil (rapeseed oil), and peanut oil. Considered safer than saturated fats.

Nucleotides: The building blocks of DNA and RNA, of which ATP is one. Nucleotides can be broken down to generate uric acid.

Omega-3 fatty acids: A type of polyunsaturated fat that is highly concentrated in foods such as fish, flaxseed, and walnuts.

Omega-6 fatty acids: A type of polyunsaturated fat found in vegetable oils such as corn oil. There are mixed reports as to whether these fats are healthy; they may have inflammatory properties.

Oxidative stress: Stress on the body from the chemical reactions of oxygen molecules, which are highly reactive. Oxidative stress is associated with inflammation and tissue damage, and is linked with increased risk for heart disease, high blood pressure, diabetes, and aging. Oxidative stress is produced during fructose metabolism and is required to activate the survival switch. Over time it can damage the mitochondria.

Polyol pathway: A series of two chemical reactions that generate fructose from glucose, in which glucose is first converted to sorbitol, which is then converted to fructose.

Polyunsaturated fat: A type of dietary fat found in many foods, but especially vegetable oils such as corn oil or safflower oil, salmon, and nuts. Polyunsaturated fats primarily comprise two types, omega-3 and omega-6 fatty acids.

Purines: Substances that are used to make DNA, ATP, and uric acid, the latter of which increases the risk of gout and metabolic syndrome. Many umami foods are rich in purines.

Satiety: The feeling of fullness.

Saturated fat: A type of dietary fat in butter, coconut oil, and fatty meats that can raise blood cholesterol levels. Saturated fats are enriched (or "saturated") in hydrogen and tend to be solid or semisolid at room temperature.

Sorbitol: A type of sugar that is part of the polyol pathway and is converted to fructose in the body. It is often used as an artificial sweetener.

Starch: Carbohydrate storage in plants that is similar to glycogen in animals. The two main types are amylose (which is digested slowly) and amylopectin (which is digested more rapidly).

Sucrose: Table sugar. Sucrose consists of a fructose and a glucose molecule bound together.

Survival switch: The noncaloric metabolic pathway activated by fructose. It is what drives development of metabolic syndrome in animals, including fat storage, insulin resistance, fatty liver, and high blood pressure. It may also have a role in other diseases, including alcoholism, cancer, and dementia.

Thrifty gene: A gene that provides survival advantages in one environment but that becomes maladaptive when in another environment. Typically, the term refers to a gene that increased the chance of survival in settings of starvation, but in settings where food is freely available may increase the risk for obesity.

Total sugars: The sugar content in a serving of a food, which includes both sugars added to the food and those normally present in the food (such as lactose in milk or fructose in apples).

Trans fats: A type of unsaturated fat typically made by partially hydrogenating (adding hydrogen to) margarine or vegetable oils to make them solid like butter or lard.

Triglycerides: The major type of fat present in our fat cells, liver, and blood. Elevated triglycerides in the blood is often observed in people who are overweight, and is considered one of the criteria of metabolic syndrome.

Trimethylamine N-oxide (TMAO): A substance that increases the risk of heart disease. It is made from red meat, largely through the actions of bacteria in the gut.

Umami: The fifth taste, also known as savory. It is the taste associated with tomato paste, Caesar salad dressing, soy, seaweed, and beer.

Uric acid: A breakdown product of purines that is generated during the metabolism of fructose and umami-rich foods. It is poorly soluble and can crystallize, especially in joints, where it causes gout, but it also has a role in driving the survival switch.

Uricase: The ancient enzyme, lost in humans, that reduces uric acid levels.

Vasopressin: A hormone released from the pituitary gland that has recently been shown to drive the development of obesity in response to sugar.

Vasopressin receptors: Vasopressin acts by binding to receptors. When it binds to the V2 receptor in the kidney, it results in the concentration of urine. However, it is the V1b receptor that is responsible for how vasopressin causes metabolic syndrome. The specific way this happens is still being figured out.

References

Introduction: The Birth of an Epidemic

Quotations

Dr. Seuss quote from *Oh, the Thinks You Can Think!* by Dr. Seuss. New York, Random House, 1975.

Sherlock Holmes quote from "The Adventure of the Priory School" by Sir Arthur Conan Doyle, *Strand Magazine*, February 1904.

Obesity and Diabetes Were Originally Rare

Johnson, R.J., Sanchez-Lozada, L.G., Andrews, P. and Lanaspa, M.A. (2017) Perspective: A historical and scientific perspective of sugar and its relation with obesity and diabetes. *Adv Nutr* 8: 412–422.

Helmchen, L.A. and Henderson, R.M. (2004) Changes in the distribution of body mass index of white US men, 1890–2000. *Ann Hum Biol* 31: 174–181.

Osler, W. (1893). *The Principles and Practice of Medicine*. New York, D. Appleton and Co.

Janeway, T.C. (1907). *The Clinical Study of Blood Pressure*. New York, D. Appleton and Co.

Emerson, H. and Larimore, L.D. (1924) Diabetes mellitus: A contribution to its epidemiology based chiefly on mortality statistics. *Arch Intern Med* 34: 585–630.

Johnson, R.J. (2012). *The Fat Switch*. Hoffman Estates, mercola.com.

Rise in Obesity in the Twentieth Century

Johnson, R.J., Perez-Pozo, S.E., Sautin, Y.Y., Manitius, J., Sanchez-Lozada, L.G., Feig, D.I., Shafiu, M., Segal, M., Glassock, R.J., Shimada, M., Roncal, C. and Nakagawa, T. (2009) Hypothesis: could excessive fructose intake and uric acid cause type 2 diabetes? *Endocr Rev* 30: 96–116.

Johnson, R.J., Sanchez-Lozada, L.G., Andrews, P. and Lanaspa, M.A. (2017) Perspective: A historical and scientific perspective of sugar and its relation with obesity and diabetes. *Adv Nutr* 8: 412–422.

Johnson, R.J., Segal, M.S., Sautin, Y., Nakagawa, T., Feig, D.I., Kang, D.H., Gersch, M.S., Benner, S. and Sanchez-Lozada, L.G. (2007) Potential role of sugar (fructose) in the epidemic of hypertension, obesity and the metabolic syndrome, diabetes, kidney disease, and cardiovascular disease. *Am J Clin Nutr* 86: 899–906.

Johnson, R.J., Titte, S., Cade, J.R., Rideout, B.A. and Oliver, W.J. (2005) Uric acid, evolution and primitive cultures. *Semin Nephrol* 25: 3–8.

Mozaffarian D., Benjamin, E.J., Go, A.S., et al. (2016) Heart disease and stroke statistics—2016 update: a report from the American Heart Association. *Circulation* 133: e38–360.

PART I: WHY NATURE WANTS US TO BE FAT

Chapter 1: The Power of Fat

Obesity in Animals as an Energy Source

Johnson, R.J., Stenvinkel, P., Martin, S.L., Jani, A., Sanchez-Lozada, L.G., Hill, J.O. and Lanaspa, M.A. (2013) Redefining metabolic syndrome as a fat storage condition based on studies of comparative physiology. *Obesity (Silver Spring)* 21: 659–664.

Bairlein, F. (2002) How to get fat: nutritional mechanisms of seasonal fat accumulation in migratory songbirds. *Naturwissenschaften* 89: 1–10.

Junk, W.J. (1985) Temporary fat storage, an adaptation of some fish species to the waterlevel fluctuations and related environmental changes of the Amazon river. *Amazoniana* 9: 315–351.

Stenvinkel, P., Jani, A.H. and Johnson, R.J. (2013) Hibernating bears (Ursidae): metabolic magicians of define interest for the nephrologist. *Kidney Int* 83: 207–212.

Stenvinkel, P., Frobert, O., Anderstam, B., Palm, F., Eriksson, M., Bragfors-Helin, A.C., Qureshi, A.R., Larsson, T., Friebe, A., Zedrosser, A., Josefsson, J., Svensson, M., Sahdo, B., Bankir, L. and Johnson, R.J. (2013) Metabolic changes in summer active and anuric hibernating free-ranging brown bears (Ursus arctos). *PLoS One* 8: e72934.

Nelson, R.A. (1973) Winter sleep in the black bear. A physiologic and metabolic marvel. *Mayo Clin Proc* 48: 733–737.

Landys, M.M., Piersma, T., Guglielmo, C.G., Jukema, J., Ramenofsky, M. and Wingfield, J.C. (2005) Metabolic profile of long-distance migratory flight and stopover in a shorebird. *Proc Biol Sci* 272: 295–302.

Johnson, R.J. (2012). *The Fat Switch*. Hoffman Estates, mercola.com.

Fasting Studies

Stewart, W.K. and Fleming, L.W. (1973) Features of a successful therapeutic fast of 382 days' duration. *Postgrad Med J* 49: 203–209.

Thomson, T.J., Runcie, J. and Miller, V. (1966) Treatment of obesity by total fasting for up to 249 days. *Lancet* 2: 992–996.

Drenick, E.J., Swendseid, M.E., Blahd, W.H. and Tuttle, S.G. (1964) Prolonged starvation as treatment for severe obesity. *JAMA* 187: 100–105.

Mildly Overweight Individuals Live Longer

Afzal, S., Tybjaerg-Hansen, A., Jensen, G.B. and Nordestgaard, B.G. (2016) Change in body mass index associated with lowest mortality in Denmark, 1976–2013. *JAMA* 315: 1989–1996.

Strulov Shachar, S. and Williams, G.R. (2017) The obesity paradox in cancer—moving beyond BMI. *Cancer Epidemiol Biomarkers Prev* 26: 13–16.

Flicker, L., McCaul, K.A., Hankey, G.J., Jamrozik, K., Brown, W.J., Byles, J.E. and Almeida, O.P. (2010) Body mass index and survival in men and women aged 70 to 75. *J Am Geriatr Soc* 58: 234–241.

Fat and Pregnancy

Frisch, R.E. (1997) Critical fatness hypothesis. *Am J Physiol* 273: E231–232.

Frisch, R.E., Wyshak, G. and Vincent, L. (1980) Delayed menarche and amenorrhea in ballet dancers. *N Engl J Med* 303: 17–19.

Frisch, R.E. (1978) Menarche and fatness: reexamination of the critical body composition hypothesis. *Science* 200: 1509–1513.

Stein, Z. and Susser, M. (1975) Fertility, fecundity, famine: food rations in the Dutch famine 1944/5 have a causal relation to fertility, and probably to fecundity. *Hum Biol* 47: 131–154.

Stein, Z. and Susser, M. (1975) The Dutch famine, 1944–1945, and the reproductive process. I. Effects on six indices at birth. *Pediatr Res* 9: 70–76.

Caloric Restriction and Longevity

Sohal, R.S. and Weindruch, R. (1996) Oxidative stress, caloric restriction, and aging. *Science* 273: 59–63.

Nisoli, E., Tonello, C., Cardile, A., Cozzi, V., Bracale, R., Tedesco, L., Falcone, S., Valerio, A., Cantoni, O., Clementi, E., Moncada, S. and Carruba, M.O. (2005) Calorie restriction promotes mitochondrial biogenesis by inducing the expression of eNOS. *Science* 310: 314–317.

Kagawa, Y. (1978) Impact of Westernization on the nutrition of Japanese: changes in physique, cancer, longevity and centenarians. *Prev Med.* 7:205–217.

Heilbronn, L.K. and Ravussin, E. (2003) Calorie restriction and aging: review of the literature and implications for studies in humans. *Am J Clin Nutr.* Sep;78:361–369.

Venus Figurines and Obesity

Johnson, R.J., Lanaspa-Garcia, M.A. and Fox, J.W. (2021) Perspective: Upper Paleolithic figurines showing women with obesity may represent survival symbols of climatic change. *Obesity (Silver Spring)* 29:11–15.

Holt, B.M. and Formicola, V. (2008) Hunters of the Ice Age: The biology of Upper Paleolithic people. *Am J Phys Anthropol* Suppl 47: 70–99.

Maier, A. and Zimmermann, A. (2017) Populations headed south? The Gravettian from a palaeodemographic point of view. *Antiquity* 91: 573–588.

Obesity and Beauty
Speke, J.H. (1864) *Journal of Discovery of the Source of the Nile.* London, Blackwood and Sons.
Darwin, C. (1871) *The Descent of Man, and Selection in Relation to Sex.* London, John Murray.
Wadd, W. (1816) *Cursory Remarks on Corpulence or Obesity Considered as a Disease with Critical Examination of Ancient and Modern Opinions Relative to the Causes and Cure.* London, Smith and Davy.

Chapter 2: Secret Reasons It Helps to Be Fat

Water Shortage and Climate Change
Kummu, M., Ward, P.J., de Moel, H. and Varis, O. (2010) Is physical water scarcity a new phenomenon? Global assessment of water shortage over the last two millennia. *Environ Res Lett* 5: 034006 (034010pp).
Fischer, E. and Knutti, R. (2015) Anthropogenic contribution to global occurrence of heavy-precipitation and high-temperature extremes. *Nature Clim Change* 5: 560–564.

Fat as a Source of Metabolic Water
Johnson, R.J., Stenvinkel, P., Jensen, T., Lanaspa, M.A., Roncal, C., Song, Z., Bankir, L. and Sanchez-Lozada, L.G. (2016) Metabolic and kidney diseases in the setting of climate change, water shortage, and survival factors. *J Am Soc Nephrol* 27: 2247–2256.
Ortiz, R.M. (2001) Osmoregulation in marine mammals. *J Exp Biol* 204: 1831–1844.
Schmidt-Nielsen, K. (1959) The physiology of the camel. *Sci Am* 201: 140–151.
Williams, J.B., Ostrowski, S., Bedin, E., Ismail, K. (2001) Seasonal variation in energy expenditure, water flux and food consumption of Arabian oryx Oryx leucoryx. *J Exp Biol.* 204 (Pt 13): 2301–2311.

Weight Is Normally Tightly Regulated
Keesey, R.E. and Hirvonen, M.D. (1997) Body weight set-points: determination and adjustment. *J Nutr* 127: 1875S–1883S.
Bessesen, D.H. (2011) Regulation of body weight: what is the regulated parameter? *Physiol Behav.* 104: 599–607.

Storing Fat Is Associated with Metabolic Syndrome in Animals and Works Like a Switch
Johnson, R.J., Stenvinkel, P., Martin, S.L., Jani, A., Sanchez-Lozada, L.G., Hill, J.O. and Lanaspa, M.A. (2013) Redefining metabolic syndrome as a fat storage condition based on studies of comparative physiology. *Obesity (Silver Spring)* 21: 659–664.
Rigano, K.S., Gehring, J.L., Evans Hutzenbiler, B.D., Chen, A.V., Nelson, O.L., Vella, C.A., Robbins, C.T. and Jansen, H.T. (2017) Life in the fat lane: seasonal regulation of insulin sensitivity, food intake, and adipose biology in brown bears. *J Comp Physiol B* 187: 649–676.

Reaven, G.M. (1999) Insulin resistance, the key to survival: a rose by any other name. *Diabetologia* 42: 384–385.

Sprengell, M., Kubera, B., Peters, A. (2021) Brain more resistant to energy restriction than body: a systematic review. *Front Neurosci.* 15: 639617.

The Overnutrition Hypothesis

Joslin, E.P., Dublin, L.I. and Marks, H.H. (1934) Studies in Diabetes mellitus. II. Its incidence and the factors underlying its variations. *Am J Med Sci* 187: 433–457.

Gortmaker, S.L., Must, A., Sobol, A.M., Peterson, K., Colditz, G.A. and Dietz, W.H. (1996) Television viewing as a cause of increasing obesity among children in the United States, 1986–1990. *Arch Pediatr Adolesc Med* 150: 356–362.

Austin, G.I., Ogden, L.G. and Hill, J.O. (2010) Trends in carbohydrate, fat, and protein intake and association with energy intake in normal-weight, overweight, and obese individuals: 1971–2006. *Am J Clin Nutr* 93: 836–843.

Evidence for a Biological Switch

Friedman, J.M. (2000) Obesity in the new millennium. *Nature* 404: 632–634.

Sahu, A. (2003) Leptin signaling in the hypothalamus: emphasis on energy homeostasis and leptin resistance. *Front Neuroendocrinol* 24: 225–253.

Robinson, T.N. (1999) Reducing children's television viewing to prevent obesity: a randomized controlled trial. *JAMA* 282: 1561–1567.

Mrosovsky, N. and Sherry, D.F. (1980) Animal anorexias. *Science* 207: 837–842.

Chapter 3: The Survival Switch

Fructose Is Used by Animals to Gain Weight

Johnson, R.J. (2012). *The Fat Switch*. Hoffman Estates, mercola.com.

Davis, D.E. (1976) Hibernation and circannual rhythms of food consumption in marmots and ground squirrels. *Q Rev Biol* 51: 477–514.

Hargrove, J.L. (2005) Adipose energy stores, physical work, and the metabolic syndrome: lessons from hummingbirds. *Nutr J* 4: 36.

Hartman, F.A. and Brownell, K.A. (1959) Liver lipids in hummingbirds. *The Condor* 61: 270–277.

Knott, C.D. (1998) Changes in orangutan caloric intake, energy balance, and ketones in response to fluctuating fruit availability. *Int J Primatol* 19: 1061–1079.

Early Studies on Fructose

Hill, R., Baker, N., Chaikoff, I.L. (1954) Altered metabolic patterns induced in the normal rat by feeding an adequate diet containing fructose as sole carbohydrate. *J Biol Chem.* 209(2): 705–716.

Bray, G.A., Nielsen, S.J. and Popkin, B.M. (2004) Consumption of high-fructose corn syrup in beverages may play a role in the epidemic of obesity. *Am J Clin Nutr* 79: 537–543.

Atkins, R. (1998). *Dr. Atkins' New Diet Revolution*. New York, Avon Books.

Elliott, S.S., Keim, N.L., Stern, J.S., Teff, K. and Havel, P.J. (2002) Fructose, weight gain, and the insulin resistance syndrome. *Am J Clin Nutr.* 76: 911–922.

Ackerman, Z., Oron-Herman, M., Grozovski, M., Rosenthal, T., Pappo, O., Link, G. and Sela, B.A. (2005) Fructose-induced fatty liver disease: hepatic effects of blood pressure and plasma triglyceride reduction. *Hypertension* 45: 1012–1018.

Sugar and HFCS

Ventura, E.E., Davis, J.N., Goran, M.I. (2011) Sugar content of popular sweetened beverages based on objective laboratory analysis: focus on fructose content. *Obesity (Silver Spring)* 19(4): 868–874.

Key Human Studies

Stanhope, K.L., Schwarz, J.M., Keim, N.L., Griffen, S.C., Bremer, A.A., Graham, J.L., Hatcher, B., Cox, C.L., Dyachenko, A., Zhang, W., McGahan, J.P., Seibert, A., Krauss, R.M., Chiu, S., Schaefer, E.J., Ai, M., Otokozawa, S., Nakajima, K., Nakano, T., Beysen, C., Hellerstein, M.K., Berglund, L. and Havel, P.J. (2009) Consuming fructose-sweetened, not glucose-sweetened, beverages increases visceral adiposity and lipids and decreases insulin sensitivity in overweight/obese humans. *J Clin Invest* 119: 1322–1334.

Perez-Pozo, S.E., Schold, J., Nakagawa, T., Sanchez-Lozada, L.G., Johnson, R.J. and Lillo, J.L. (2010) Excessive fructose intake induces the features of metabolic syndrome in healthy adult men: role of uric acid in the hypertensive response. *Int J Obes (Lond)* 34: 454–461.

Cox, C.L., Stanhope, K.L., Schwarz, J.M., Graham, J.L., Hatcher, B., Griffen, S.C., Bremer, A.A., Berglund, L., McGahan, J.P., Havel, P.J. and Keim, N.L. (2012) Consumption of fructose-sweetened beverages for 10 weeks reduces net fat oxidation and energy expenditure in overweight/obese men and women. *Eur J Clin Nutr* 66: 201–208.

Fructose Causes Metabolic Syndrome in Animals: Mechanisms

Role of Uric Acid

Nakagawa, T., Tuttle, K.R., Short, R.A. and Johnson, R.J. (2005) Hypothesis: fructose-induced hyperuricemia as a causal mechanism for the epidemic of the metabolic syndrome. *Nat Clin Pract Nephrol* 1: 80–86.

Nakagawa, T., Hu, H., Zharikov, S., Tuttle, K.R., Short, R.A., Glushakova, O., Ouyang, X., Feig, D.I., Block, E.R., Herrera-Acosta, J., Patel, J.M. and Johnson, R.J. (2006) A causal role for uric acid in fructose-induced metabolic syndrome. *Am J Physiol Renal Physiol* 290: F625–631.

Role of Calories

Roncal-Jimenez, C.A., Lanaspa, M.A., Rivard, C.J., Nakagawa, T., Sanchez-Lozada, L.G., Jalal, D., Andres-Hernando, A., Tanabe, K., Madero, M., Li, N., Cicerchi, C., McFann, K., Sautin, Y.Y. and Johnson, R.J. (2011) Sucrose induces fatty liver and pancreatic inflammation in male breeder rats independent of excess energy intake. *Metabolism* 60: 1259–1270.

Reungjui S., Roncal C.A., Mu W., Srinivas T.R., Sirivongs D., Johnson R.J., and Nakagawa T. (2007) Thiazide diuretics exacerbate fructose-induced metabolic syndrome. *J Am Soc Nephrol.* 18: 2724–2731.

Role of Leptin
Shapiro, A., Mu, W., Roncal, C., Cheng, K.Y., Johnson, R.J. and Scarpace, P.J. (2008) Fructose-induced leptin resistance exacerbates weight gain in response to subsequent high-fat feeding. *Am J Physiol Regul Integr Comp Physiol* 295: R1370–1375.
Shapiro, A., Tumer, N., Gao, Y., Cheng, K.Y. and Scarpace, P.J. (2011) Prevention and reversal of diet-induced leptin resistance with a sugar-free diet despite high fat content. *Br J Nutr* 106: 390–397.

Role of Taste
de Araujo, I.E., Oliveira-Maia, A.J., Sotnikova, T.D., Gainetdinov, R.R., Caron, M.G., Nicolelis, M.A., and Simon, S.A. (2008) Food reward in the absence of taste receptor signaling. *Neuron* 57(6): 930–941.
Andres-Hernando, A., Kuwabara, M., Orlicky, D.J., Vandenbeuch, A., Cicerchi, C., Kinnamon, S.C., Finger, T.E., Johnson, R.J. and Lanaspa, M.A. (2020) Sugar causes obesity and metabolic syndrome in mice independently of sweet taste. *Am J Physiol Endocrinol Metab* 319: E276–E290.

Role of Metabolism
Ishimoto, T., Lanaspa, M.A., Le, M.T., Garcia, G.E., Diggle, C.P., Maclean, P.S., Jackman, M.R., Asipu, A., Roncal-Jimenez, C.A., Kosugi, T., Rivard, C.J., Maruyama, S., Rodriguez-Iturbe, B., Sanchez-Lozada, L.G., Bonthron, D.T., Sautin, Y.Y. and Johnson, R.J. (2012) Opposing effects of fructokinase C and A isoforms on fructose-induced metabolic syndrome in mice. *Proc Natl Acad Sci U S A* 109: 4320–4325.
Softic, S., Gupta, M.K., Wang, G.X., Fujisaka, S., O'Neill, B.T., Rao, T.N., Willoughby, J., Harbison, C., Fitzgerald, K., Ilkayeva, O., Newgard, C.B., Cohen, D.E. and Kahn, C.R. (2018) Divergent effects of glucose and fructose on hepatic lipogenesis and insulin signaling. *J Clin Invest* 128: 1199.
Miller, C.O., Yang, X., Lu, K., Cao, J., Herath, K., Rosahl, T.W., Askew, R., Pavlovic, G., Zhou, G., Li, C. and Akiyama, T.E. (2018) Ketohexokinase knockout mice, a model for essential fructosuria, exhibit altered fructose metabolism and are protected from diet-induced metabolic defects. *Am J Physiol Endocrinol Metab* 315(3): E386–E393.

Separating Craving and Metabolic Syndrome
Andres-Hernando, A., Orlicky, D.J., Kuwabara, M., Ishimoto, T., Nakagawa, T., Johnson, R.J. and Lanaspa, M.A. (2020) Deletion of fructokinase in the liver or in the intestine reveals differential effects on sugar-induced metabolic dysfunction. *Cell Metab* 32(1): 117–127

How the Switch Works

ATP Depletion, Oxidative Stress, and Altered Mitochondrial Function

Maenpaa, P.H., Raivio, K.O. and Kekomaki, M.P. (1968) Liver adenine nucleotides: fructose-induced depletion and its effect on protein synthesis. *Science* 161: 1253–1254.

Bawden, S.J., Stephenson, M.C., Ciampi, E., Hunter, K., Marciani, L., Macdonald, I.A., Aithal, G.P., Morris, P.G. and Gowland, P.A. (2016) Investigating the effects of an oral fructose challenge on hepatic ATP reserves in healthy volunteers: A (31)P MRS study. *Clin Nutr* 35: 645–649.

Lanaspa, M.A., Cicerchi, C., Garcia, G., Li, N., Roncal-Jimenez, C.A., Rivard, C.J., Hunter, B., Andres-Hernando, A., Ishimoto, T., Sanchez-Lozada, L.G., Thomas, J., Hodges, R.S., Mant, C.T. and Johnson, R.J. (2012) Counteracting Roles of AMP Deaminase and AMP Kinase in the Development of Fatty Liver. *PLoS ONE* 7: e48801.

Lanaspa, M.A., Sanchez-Lozada, L.G., Choi, Y.J., Cicerchi, C., Kanbay, M., Roncal-Jimenez, C.A., Ishimoto, T., Li, N., Marek, G., Duranay, M., Schreiner, G., Rodriguez-Iturbe, B., Nakagawa, T., Kang, D.H., Sautin, Y.Y. and Johnson, R.J. (2012) Uric acid induces hepatic steatosis by generation of mitochondrial oxidative stress: potential role in fructose-dependent and -independent fatty liver. *J Biol Chem* 287: 40732–40744.

Softic, S., Meyer, J.G., Wang, G.X., Gupta, M.K., Batista, T.M., Lauritzen, H., Fujisaka, S., Serra, D., Herrero, L., Willoughby, J., Fitzgerald, K., Ilkayeva, O., Newgard, C.B., Gibson, B.W., Schilling, B., Cohen, D.E. and Kahn, C.R. (2019) Dietary sugars alter hepatic fatty acid oxidation via transcriptional and post-translational modifications of mitochondrial proteins. *Cell Metab* 30: 735–753 e734.

Softic, S., Stanhope, K.L., Boucher, J., Divanovic, S., Lanaspa, M.A., Johnson, R.J. and Kahn, C.R. (2020) Fructose and hepatic insulin resistance. *Crit Rev Clin Lab Sci* 57: 1–15.

Johnson, R.J., Nakagawa, T., Sanchez-Lozada, L.G., Shafiu, M., Sundaram, S., Le, M., Ishimoto, T., Sautin, Y.Y. and Lanaspa, M.A. (2013) Sugar, uric acid, and the etiology of diabetes and obesity. *Diabetes* 62: 3307–3315.

Johnson, R.J. (2012). *The Fat Switch*. Hoffman Estates, mercola.com.

Chapter 4: Why We Are Becoming Fat

Orangutan Use Fruit to Gain Fat

Knott, C.D. (1998) Changes in orangutan caloric intake, energy balance, and ketones in response to fluctuating fruit availability. *Int J Primatol* 19: 1061–1079.

Vitamin C Mutation and the Extinction of the Dinosaurs

Tavare, S., Marshall, C.R., Will, O., Soligo, C. and Martin, R.D. (2002) Using the fossil record to estimate the age of the last common ancestor of extant primates. *Nature* 416: 726–729.

Pozzi, L., Hodgson, J.A., Burrell, A.S., Sterner, K.N., Raaum, R.L. and Disotell, T.R. (2014) Primate phylogenetic relationships and divergence dates inferred from complete mitochondrial genomes. *Mol Phylogenet Evol* 75: 165–183.

Schulte, P., Alegret, L., Arenillas, I., et al. (2010) The Chicxulub asteroid impact and mass extinction at the Cretaceous-Paleogene boundary. *Science* 327: 1214–1218.

Vellekoop, J., Sluijs, A., Smit, J., Schouten, S., Weijers, J.W., Sinninghe Damste, J.S. and Brinkhuis, H. (2014) Rapid short-term cooling following the Chicxulub impact at the Cretaceous-Paleogene boundary. *Proc Natl Acad Sci U S A* 111: 7537–7541.

Johnson, R.J., Gaucher, E.A., Sautin, Y.Y., Henderson, G.N., Angerhofer, A.J. and Benner, S.A. (2008) The planetary biology of ascorbate and uric acid and their relationship with the epidemic of obesity and cardiovascular disease. *Med Hypotheses* 71: 22–31.

Uricase Mutation and the Thrifty Gene Hypothesis

Neel, J.V. (1962) Diabetes mellitus: a "thrifty" genotype rendered detrimental by "progress"? *Am J Hum Genet* 14: 353–362.

Andrews, P. (2015) *An Ape's View of Human Evolution.* Cambridge, Cambridge University Press.

Cohen, R. (August 2013) Sugar love: a not so sweet story. *National Geographic*: 79–97.

Johnson, R.J. and Andrews, P. (2015) The fat gene: A genetic mutation in prehistoric apes may underlie today's pandemic of obesity and diabetes. *Scientific American* 313: 64–69.

Andrews, P. and Kelley, J. (2007) Middle Miocene dispersals of apes. *Folia Primatol (Basel)* 78: 328–343.

Begun, D.R. (2000) Middle Miocene hominoid origins. *Science* 287: 2375.

Johnson, R.J. and Andrews, P. (2010) Fructose, uricase, and the back-to-Africa hypothesis. *Evol Anthropol* 19: 250–257.

Kratzer, J.T., Lanaspa, M.A., Murphy, M.N., Cicerchi, C., Graves, C.L., Tipton, P.A., Ortlund, E.A., Johnson, R.J. and Gaucher, E.A. (2014) Evolutionary history and metabolic insights of ancient mammalian uricases. *Proc Natl Acad Sci U S A* 111: 3763–3768.

Johnson, R.J., Titte, S., Cade, J.R., Rideout, B.A. and Oliver, W.J. (2005) Uric acid, evolution and primitive cultures. *Semin Nephrol* 25: 3–8.

Johnson, R.J., Stenvinkel, P., Andrews, P., Sanchez-Lozada, L.G., Nakagawa, T., Gaucher, E., Andres-Hernando, A., Rodriguez-Iturbe, B., Jimenez, C.R., Garcia, G., Kang, D.H., Tolan, D.R. and Lanaspa, M.A. (2020) Fructose metabolism as a common evolutionary pathway of survival associated with climate change, food shortage and droughts. *J Intern Med* 287: 252–262.

Cavities as a Sign of Fructose Exposure

Hujoel, P. (2009) Dietary carbohydrates and dental-systemic diseases. *J Dent Res* 88: 490–502.

Burne, R.A., Chen, Y.Y., Wexler, D.L., Kuramitsu, H. and Bowen, W.H. (1996) Cariogenicity of Streptococcus mutans strains with defects in fructan metabolism assessed in a program-fed specific-pathogen-free rat model. *J Dent Res* 75: 1572–1577.

Obesity in Ancient Egypt

Saleem, S.N. and Hawass, Z. (2014) Ankylosing spondylitis or diffuse idiopathic skeletal hyperostosis in royal Egyptian mummies of 18th–20th Dynasties? CT and archaeology studies. *Arthritis Rheumatol* 66: 3311–3316.

Breasted, J.H. (1906) *Ancient Records of Egypt: The Eighteenth Dynasty*. Chicago, University of Chicago Press.

The History of Sugar
Mintz, S. (1986) *Sweetness and Power*. New York: Penguin Books.

Deer N. (1949–50) *The History of Sugar*. London: Chapman and Hall.

Bhishagranta, K.K.L. (1907) *An English Translation of the Sushruta Samhita*. Calcutta, Mihir Press.

Rosner, F. (2002) The Life of Moses Maimonides, a Prominent Medieval Physician. *Einstein Quart J Biol Med* 19: 125–128.

Austen, R.A. and Smith, W.D. (1990) Private tooth decay as public economic virtue: The slave: sugar triangle, consumerism, and European industrialization. *Social Science History* 14: 95–115.

Smith, W.D. (1992) Complications of the commonplace: Tea, sugar and imperialism. *J Interdisciplinary History* 23: 259–278.

Rivard, C., Thomas, J., Lanaspa, M.A. and Johnson, R.J. (2013) Sack and sugar, and the aetiology of gout in England between 1650 and 1900. *Rheumatology (Oxford)* 52: 421–426.

Sugar. *The Penny Cyclopaedia of the Society for the Diffusion of Useful Knowledge*, Lord Brougham, ed. Charles Knight and Co, London, 1842, vol 23, pp 224–238.

Watts, W. (1848) On the symptoms, varieties, and remote causes of diabetes. *The Lancet* 51; 439–441 and 661–663.

Wadd, W. (1816) *Cursory remarks on corpulence or obesity considered as a disease with critical examination of ancient and modern opinions relative to the causes and cure*. Smith and Davy, London.

The Effect of Sugar on Minorities
Diamond, J. (2003) The double puzzle of diabetes. *Nature* 423: 599–602.

Christie, T. (1811) Notes on diabetes mellitus, as it occurs in Ceylon. *Edinb Med Surg J.* 7: 285–299.

Saab, K.R., Kendrick, J., Yracheta, J.M., Lanaspa, M.A., Pollard, M. and Johnson, R.J. (2015) New insights on the risk for cardiovascular disease in African Americans: the role of added sugars. *J Am Soc Nephrol* 26: 247–257.

Johnson, R.J., Lanaspa, M.A., Sanchez-Lozada, L.G., Rivard, C.J., Rodriguez-Iturbe, B., Merriman, T.R. and Sundborn, G. (2014) Fat storage syndrome in Pacific peoples: a combination of environment and genetics? *Public Health Dialogue* 20: 11–16.

Yracheta, J.M., Alfonso, J., Lanaspa, M.A., Roncal-Jimenez, C., Johnson, S.B., Sanchez-Lozada, L.G. and Johnson, R.J. (2015) Hispanic Americans living in the United States and their risk for obesity, diabetes and kidney disease: Genetic and environmental considerations. *Postgrad Med* 127: 503–510.

Yracheta, J.M., Lanaspa, M.A., Le, M.T., Abdelmalak, M.F., Alfonso, J., Sanchez-Lozada, L.G. and Johnson, R.J. (2015) Diabetes and kidney disease in American Indians: potential role of sugar-sweetened beverages. *Mayo Clin Proc* 90: 813–823.

Sugar Consumption Is Decreasing and Is Associated with Slowing of the Obesity and Diabetes Epidemics

Statistical Abstract of the United States, 2011. Table 217. United States Census Bureau, https://www.census.gov/library/publications/2011/compendia/statab/131ed.html.

Geiss, L.S., Wang, J., Cheng, Y.J., Thompson, T.J., Barker, L., Li, Y., Albright, A.L. and Gregg, E.W. (2014) Prevalence and incidence trends for diagnosed diabetes among adults aged 20 to 79 years, United States, 1980–2012. *JAMA* 312: 1218–1226.

Flegal, K.M., Carroll, M.D., Kit, B.K. and Ogden CL. (2012) Prevalence of obesity and trends in the distribution of body mass index among US adults, 1999–2010. *JAMA* 307: 491–497.

The Effect of Fructose (or Sucrose) on Human Metabolic Syndrome

Stanhope, K.L., Schwarz, J.M., Keim, N.L., Griffen, S.C., Bremer, A.A., Graham, J.L., Hatcher, B., Cox, C.L., Dyachenko, A., Zhang, W., McGahan, J.P., Seibert, A., Krauss, R.M., Chiu, S., Schaefer, E.J., Ai, M., Otokozawa, S., Nakajima, K., Nakano, T., Beysen, C., Hellerstein, M.K., Berglund, L. and Havel, P.J. (2009) Consuming fructose-sweetened, not glucose-sweetened, beverages increases visceral adiposity and lipids and decreases insulin sensitivity in overweight/obese humans. *J Clin Invest* 119: 1322–1334.

Perez-Pozo, S.E., Schold, J., Nakagawa, T., Sánchez-Lozada, L.G., Johnson, R.J. and Lillo, J.L. (2010) Excessive fructose intake induces the features of metabolic syndrome in healthy adult men: role of uric acid in the hypertensive response. *Int J Obes (Lond)* 34: 454–461.

Maersk, M., Belza, A., Stødkilde-Jørgensen, H., Ringgaard, S., Chabanova, E., Thomsen, H., Pedersen, S.B., Astrup, A. and Richelsen, B. (2012) Sucrose-sweetened beverages increase fat storage in the liver, muscle, and visceral fat depot: a 6-mo randomized intervention study. *Am J Clin Nutr* 95: 283–289.

Lustig, R.H., Mulligan, K., Noworolski, S.M., Tai, V.W., Wen, M.J., Erkin-Cakmak, A., Gugliucci, A. and Schwarz, J.M. (2016) Isocaloric fructose restriction and metabolic improvement in children with obesity and metabolic syndrome. *Obesity (Silver Spring)* 24: 453–460.

Schwimmer, J.B., Ugalde-Nicalo, P., Welsh, J.A., Angeles, J.E., Cordero, M., Harlow, K.E., Alazraki, A., Durelle, J., Knight-Scott, J., Newton, K.P., Cleeton, R., Knott, C., Konomi, J., Middleton, M.S., Travers, C., Sirlin, C.B., Hernandez, A., Sekkarie, A., McCracken, C. and Vos, M.B. (2019) Effect of a low free sugar diet vs usual diet on nonalcoholic fatty liver disease in adolescent boys: a randomized clinical trial. *JAMA* 321: 256–265.

Chapter 5: An Unpleasant Surprise: It's Not Just Fructose

A Low-Fructose Diet to Cure Obesity

Johnson, R.J. (with Tim Gower). (2008) *The Sugar Fix. The High-Fructose Fallout That Is Making You Fat and Sick*. New York, Rodale Press.

The Polyol Pathway and the Production of Fructose from Glucose

Andres-Hernando, A., Johnson, R.J. and Lanaspa, M.A. (2019) Endogenous fructose production: what do we know and how relevant is it? *Curr Opin Clin Nutr Metab Care* 22: 289–294.

Lanaspa, M.A., Ishimoto, T., Li, N., Cicerchi, C., Orlicky, D.J., Ruzycki, P., Rivard, C., Inaba, S., Roncal-Jimenez, C.A., Bales, E.S., Diggle, C.P., Asipu, A., Petrash, J.M., Kosugi, T., Maruyama, S., Sanchez-Lozada, L.G., McManaman, J.L., Bonthron, D.T., Sautin, Y.Y. and Johnson, R.J. (2013) Endogenous fructose production and metabolism in the liver contributes to the development of metabolic syndrome. *Nat Commun* 4: 2434.

Andres-Hernando, A., Orlicky, D.J., Kuwabara, M., Ishimoto, T., Nakagawa, T., Johnson, R.J. and Lanaspa, M.A. (2020) Deletion of fructokinase in the liver or in the intestine reveals differential effects on sugar-induced metabolic dysfunction. *Cell Metab* 32(1): 117–127.

Francey, C., Cros, J., Rosset, R., Creze, C., Rey, V., Stefanoni, N., Schneiter, P., Tappy, L. and Seyssel, K. (2019) The extra-splanchnic fructose escape after ingestion of a fructose-glucose drink: An exploratory study in healthy humans using a dual fructose isotope method. *Clin Nutr ESPEN* 29: 125–132.

High-Glycemic Carbohydrates and Obesity

Taubes, G. (2007) *Good Calories, Bad Calories.* New York, Alfred A. Knopf.

Ludwig, D.S. and Ebbeling, C.B. (2018) The carbohydrate-insulin model of obesity: beyond "calories in, calories out." *JAMA Intern Med* 178: 1098–1103.

Amylase and Genetics

Patin, E. and Quintana-Murci, L. (2008) Demeter's legacy: rapid changes to our genome imposed by diet. *Trends Ecol Evol* 23: 56–59.

Perry, G.H., Dominy, N.J., Claw, K.G., Lee, A.S., Fiegler, H., Redon, R., Werner, J., Villanea, F.A., Mountain, J.L., Misra, R., Carter, N.P., Lee, C. and Stone, A.C. (2007) Diet and the evolution of human amylase gene copy number variation. *Nat Genet* 39: 1256–1260.

Dehydration and Salt

Joyce, J.P. and Brunswick, C.F. (1975) Sodium supplementation of sheep and cattle fed lucerne. *New Zealand Journal of Experimental Agriculture* 3: 299–304.

Lanaspa, M.A., Kuwabara, M., Andres-Hernando, A., Li, N., Cicerchi, C., Jensen, T., Orlicky, D.J., Roncal-Jimenez, C.A., Ishimoto, T., Nakagawa, T., Rodriguez-Iturbe, B., MacLean, P.S. and Johnson, R.J. (2018) High salt intake causes leptin resistance and obesity in mice by stimulating endogenous fructose production and metabolism. *Proc Natl Acad Sci U S A* 115: 3138–3143.

Donovan, D.S., Solomon, C.G., Seely, E.W., Williams, G.H. and Simonson, D.C. (1993) Effect of sodium intake on insulin sensitivity. *Am J Physiol.* 264(5 Pt 1): E730–734.

Libuda, L., Kersting, M. and Alexy, U. (2012) Consumption of dietary salt measured by urinary sodium excretion and its association with body weight status in healthy children and adolescents. *Public Health Nutr* 15: 433–441.

Larsen, S.C., Ängquist, L., Sørensen, T.I. and Heitmann, B.L. (2013) 24h urinary sodium excretion and subsequent change in weight, waist circumference and body composition. *PLoS One* 8(7): e69689.

Hu, G., Jousilahti, P., Peltonen, M., Lindström, J. and Tuomilehto, J. (2005) Urinary sodium and potassium excretion and the risk of type 2 diabetes: a prospective study in Finland. *Diabetologia* 48: 1477–1483

Stookey, J.D., Barclay, D., Arieff, A. and Popkin, B.M. (2007) The altered fluid distribution in obesity may reflect plasma hypertonicity. *Eur J Clin Nutr* 61: 190–199.

Stookey, J.D., Kavouras, S., Suh, H. and Lang, F. (2020) Underhydration is associated with obesity, chronic diseases, and death within 3 to 6 years in the U.S. population aged 51–70 Years. *Nutrients* 12 (6): 905.

Vasopressin as the Fat Hormone and the Power of Water

Andres-Hernando, A., Jensen, T.J., Kuwabara, M., Orlicky, D.J., Cicerchi, C,. Li, N., Roncal-Jimenez, C.A., Garcia, G.E., Ishimoto, T., Maclean, P.S., Bjornstad, P., Sanchez-Lozada, L.G., Kanbay, M., Nakagawa, T., Johnson, R.J. and Lanaspa, M.A. (2021) Vasopressin mediates fructose-induced metabolic syndrome by activating the V1b receptor. *JCI Insight* 6: e140848.

Enhörning, S., Bankir, L., Bouby, N., Struck, J., Hedblad, B., Persson, M., Morgenthaler, N.G., Nilsson, P.M. and Melander, O. (2013) Copeptin, a marker of vasopressin, in abdominal obesity, diabetes and microalbuminuria: the prospective Malmo Diet and Cancer Study cardiovascular cohort. *Int J Obes (Lond)* 37: 598–603.

Enhörning, S., Struck, J., Wirfalt, E., Hedblad, B., Morgenthaler, N.G. and Melander, O. (2011) Plasma copeptin, a unifying factor behind the metabolic syndrome. *J Clin Endocrinol Metab* 96: E1065–1072.

Song, Z., Roncal-Jimenez, C.A., Lanaspa-Garcia, M.A., Oppelt, S.A., Kuwabara, M., Jensen, T., Milagres, T., Andres-Hernando, A., Ishimoto, T., Garcia, G.E., Johnson, G., MacLean, P.S., Sanchez-Lozada, L.G., Tolan, D.R. and Johnson, R.J. (2017) Role of fructose and fructokinase in acute dehydration-induced vasopressin gene expression and secretion in mice. *J Neurophysiol* 117: 646–654.

Chapman, C.L., Johnson, B.D., Sackett, J.R., Parker, M.D. and Schlader, Z.J. (2019) Soft drink consumption during and following exercise in the heat elevates biomarkers of acute kidney injury. *Am J Physiol Regul Integr Comp Physiol* 316: R189–R198.

Kanbay, M., Guler, B., Ertgulu, L.A., Dagel, T., Afsar, B., Incir, S., Baygul, A., Covic, A., Andres-Hernando, A., Sanchez-Lozada, L.G., Lanaspa, M.A. and Johnson, R.J. (2021) The speed of ingestion of a sugary beverage has an effect on the acute metabolic response to fructose. *Nutrients* 3: 1916.

Bouby, N., Bachmann, S., Bichet, D. and Bankir, L. (1990) Effect of water intake on the progression of chronic renal failure in the 5/6 nephrectomized rat. *Am J Physiol* 258(4 Pt 2): F973–979.

Taveau, C., Chollet, C., Waeckel, L., Desposito, D., Bichet, D.G., Arthus, M.F., Magnan, C., Philippe, E., Paradis, V., Foufelle, F., Hainault, I., Enhörning, S., Velho, G., Roussel, R., Bankir, L., Melander, O. and Bouby, N. (2015) Vasopressin and hydration play a major role in the development of glucose intolerance and hepatic steatosis in obese rats. *Diabetologia* 58: 1081–1090.

Stookey, J.D., Constant, F., Popkin, B.M. and Gardner, C.D. (2008) Drinking water is associated with weight loss in overweight dieting women independent of diet and activity. *Obesity (Silver Spring)* 16: 2481–2488.

Enhörning, S., Brunkwall, L., Tasevska, I., Ericson, U., Persson Tholin, J., Persson, M., Lemetais, G., Vanhaecke, T., Dolci, A., Perrier, E.T. and Melander, O. (2019) Water supplementation reduces copeptin and plasma glucose in adults with high copeptin: the H_2O metabolism pilot study. *J Clin Endocrinol Metab* 104: 1917–1925.

Patel, A.I. and Hampton, K.E. (2011) Encouraging consumption of water in school and child care settings: access, challenges, and strategies for improvement. *Am J Public Health* 101: 1370–1379.

Schwartz, A.E., Leardo, M., Aneja, S. and Elbel, B. (2016) Effect of a school-based water intervention on child body mass index and obesity. *JAMA Pediatr* 170: 220–226.

Jones, S.J., Gonzalez, W. and Frongillo, E.A. (2010) Policies that restrict sweetened beverage availability may reduce consumption in elementary-school children. *Public Health Nutr* 13: 589–595.

Muckelbauer, R., Libuda, L., Clausen, K., Toschke, A.M., Reinehr, T. and Kersting, M. (2009) Promotion and provision of drinking water in schools for overweight prevention: randomized, controlled cluster trial. *Pediatrics* 123: e661–667.

Umami as a Risk Factor for Obesity

Andres-Hernando, A., Cicerchi, C., Kuwabara, M., Orlicky, D.J., Sanchez Lozada, L.G., Nakagawa, T., Johnson, R.J. and Lanaspa-Garcia, M.A. (2021) Umami-induced obesity and metabolic syndrome is mediated by nucleotide degradation and uric acid generation. *Nature Metabolism* 3: 1189–1201.

Johnson, R.J., Nakagawa, T., Sanchez-Lozada, L.G., Lanaspa, M.A., Tamura, Y., Tanabe, K., Ishimoto, T., Thomas, J., Inaba, S., Kitagawa, W. and Rivard, C.J. (2013) Umami: the taste that drives purine intake. *J Rheumatol* 40: 1794–1796.

Ninomiya, K. (1998) Natural occurrence. *Food Rev Int* 14: 177–211.

He, K., Du, S., Xun, P., Sharma, S., Wang, H., Zhai, F. and Popkin, B. (2011) Consumption of monosodium glutamate in relation to incidence of overweight in Chinese adults: China Health and Nutrition Survey (CHNS). *Am J Clin Nutr* 93: 1328–1336.

PART II: THE FAT SWITCH AND DISEASE

Chapter 6: The Bread-and-Butter Diseases of Humankind

Gout

Singh, G., Lingala, B. and Mithal A. (2019) Gout and hyperuricaemia in the USA: prevalence and trends. *Rheumatology (Oxford)* 58(12): 2177–2180.

Johnson, R.J., Bakris, G.L., Borghi, C., Chonchol, M.B., Feldman, D., Lanaspa, M.A., Merriman, T.R., Moe, O.W., Mount, D.B., Sanchez Lozada, L.G., Stahl, E., Weiner, D.E. and Chertow, G.M. (2018) Hyperuricemia, acute and chronic kidney disease, hypertension, and cardiovascular disease: report of a scientific workshop organized by the National Kidney Foundation. *Am J Kidney Dis* 71: 851–865.

Feig, D.I., Soletsky, B. and Johnson, R.J. (2008) Effect of allopurinol on blood pressure of adolescents with newly diagnosed essential hypertension: a randomized trial. *JAMA* 300(8): 924–932.

Soletsky, B. and Feig, D.I. (2012) Uric acid reduction rectifies prehypertension in obese adolescents. *Hypertension* 60: 1148–1156.

Takir, M., Kostek, O., Ozkok, A., Elcioglu, O.C., Bakan, A., Erek, A., Mutlu, H.H., Telci, O., Semerci, A., Odabas, A.R., Afsar, B., Smits, G.A., Lanaspa, M., Sharma, S., Johnson, R.J. and Kanbay, M. (2015) Lowering uric acid with allopurinol improves insulin resistance and systemic inflammation in asymptomatic hyperuricemia. *J Investig Med* 63(8): 924–929.

King, C., Lanaspa, M.A., Jensen, T., Tolan, D.R., Sánchez-Lozada, L.G. and Johnson, R.J. (2018) Uric acid as a cause of the metabolic syndrome. *Contrib Nephrol* 192: 88–102.

Kanbay, M., Ozkara, A., Selcoki, Y., Isik, B., Turgut, F., Bavbek, N., Uz, E., Akcay, A., Yigitoglu, R. and Covic, A. (2007) Effect of treatment of hyperuricemia with allopurinol on blood pressure, creatinine clearence, and proteinuria in patients with normal renal functions. *Int Urol Nephrol* 39: 1227–1233.

Kuwabara, M., Niwa, K., Hisatome, I., Nakagawa, T., Roncal-Jimenez, C.A., Andres-Hernando, A., Bjornstad, P., Jensen, T., Sato, Y., Milagres, T., Garcia, G., Ohno, M., Lanaspa, M.A. and Johnson, R.J. (2017) Asymptomatic hyperuricemia without comorbidities predicts cardiometabolic diseases: five-year Japanese cohort study. *Hypertension.* 69: 1036–1044.

Madero, M., Rodríguez Castellanos, F.E., Jalal, D., Villalobos-Martín, M., Salazar, J., Vazquez-Rangel, A., Johnson, R.J. and Sanchez-Lozada, L.G. (2015) A pilot study on the impact of a low fructose diet and allopurinol on clinic blood pressure among overweight and prehypertensive subjects: a randomized placebo controlled trial. *J Am Soc Hypertens.* 9: 837–844.

McMullan, C.J., Borgi, L., Fisher, N., Curhan, G. and Forman, J. (2017) Effect of uric acid lowering on renin-angiotensin-system activation and ambulatory BP: a randomized controlled trial. *Clin J Am Soc Nephrol* 12: 807–816.

Klauser, A.S., Halpern, E.J., Strobl, S., Gruber, J., Feuchtner, G., Bellmann-Weiler, R., Weiss, G., Stofferin, H. and Jaschke, W. (2019) Dual-energy computed tomography detection of cardiovascular monosodium urate deposits in patients with gout. *JAMA Cardiol* 4: 1019–1028.

Khanna, P., Johnson, R.J., Marder, B., LaMoreaux, B. and Kumar, A. (2020) Systemic urate deposition: an unrecognized complication of gout? *J Clin Med* 9:(10): 3204.

Diabetes

Lancereaux, E. (1880) Le Diabete maigre et le Diabete gras. *L' Union Mid.*

Wadd, W. (1816) *Cursory Remarks on Corpulence or Obesity Considered as a Disease with Critical Examination of Ancient and Modern Opinions Relative to the Causes and Cure*. London, Smith and Davy.

Charles, R. (1907) Diabetes in the tropics. *Br Med J* 19: 1051–1064.

Emerson, H. and Larimore, L.D. (1924) Diabetes mellitus: a contribution to its epidemiology based chiefly on mortality statistics. *Arch Intern Med* 34: 585–630.

Banting, F. (1929) The history of insulin. *Edin Med J* 36: 2–6.

Mills, C.A. (1930) Diabetes mellitus: Sugar consumption in its etiology. *Arch Int Med* 30: 582–584.

Spiegelman M. and Marks H.H. (1946) Age and sex variations in the prevalence and onset of diabetes mellitus. *Am J Public Health Nation's Health* 36(1): 26–33.

Joslin, E.P., Dubin, L.I. and Marks, H.H. (1934) Studies in diabetes mellitus II. Its incidene and the factors underling its variations. *Am J Med Sci* 187: 433–457.

Malik, V.S., Popkin, B.M., Bray, G.A., Després, J.P., Willett, W.C. and Hu, F.B. (2010) Sugar-sweetened beverages and risk of metabolic syndrome and type 2 diabetes: a meta-analysis. *Diabetes Care* 33: 2477–2483.

Willett, W., Manson, J. and Liu, S. (2002) Glycemic index, glycemic load, and risk of type 2 diabetes. *Am J Clin Nutr* 76: 274S–280S.

Aeberli, I., Hochuli, M., Gerber, P.A., Sze, L., Murer, S.B., Tappy, L., Spinas, G.A. and Berneis, K. (2013) Moderate amounts of fructose consumption impair insulin sensitivity in healthy young men: a randomized controlled trial. *Diabetes Care* 36: 150–156.

Stanhope, K.L., Schwarz, J.M., Keim, N.L. et al. (2009) Consuming fructose-sweetened, not glucose-sweetened, beverages increases visceral adiposity and lipids and decreases insulin sensitivity in overweight/obese humans. *J Clin Invest* 119: 1322–1334.

Lustig, R.H., Mulligan, K., Noworolski, S.M., Tai, V.W., Wen, M.J., Erkin-Cakmak, A., Gugliucci, A. and Schwarz, JM. (2016) Isocaloric fructose restriction and metabolic improvement in children with obesity and metabolic syndrome. *Obesity (Silver Spring)* 24: 453–460.

Hu, E.A., Pan, A., Malik, V. and Sun, Q. (2012) White rice consumption and risk of type 2 diabetes: meta-analysis and systematic review. *BMJ* 344: e1454.

Muraki, I., Rimm, E.B., Willett, W.C., Manson, J.E., Hu, F.B. and Sun, Q. (2016) Potato consumption and risk of type 2 diabetes: results from three prospective cohort studies. *Diabetes Care* 39: 376–384.

Song, Y., Manson, J.E., Buring, J.E. and Liu, S. (2004) A prospective study of red meat consumption and type 2 diabetes in middle-aged and elderly women: the Women's Health Study. *Diabetes Care* 27(9): 2108–2115.

Hypertension

Brown, C.M., Dulloo, A.G., Yepuri, G. and Montani, J.P. (2008) Fructose ingestion acutely elevates blood pressure in healthy young humans. *Am J Physiol Regul Integr Comp Physiol* 294: R730–737.

Jalal, D.I., Smits, G., Johnson, R.J. and Chonchol, M. (2010) Increased fructose associates with elevated blood pressure. *J Am Soc Nephrol* 21: 1543–1549.

Kanbay, M., Aslan, G., Afsar, B., Dagel, T., Siriopol, D., Kuwabara, M., Incir, S., Camkiran, V., Rodriguez-Iturbe, B., Lanaspa, M.A., Covic, A. and Johnson, R.J. (2018) Acute effects of salt on blood pressure are mediated by serum osmolality. *J Clin Hypertens (Greenwich)* 20: 1447–1454.

Kuwabara, M., Kanbay, M., Niwa, K., Ae, R., Andres-Hernando, A., Roncal-Jimenez, C.A., Garcia, G., Sanchez-Lozada, L.G., Rodriguez-Iturbe, B., Hisatome, I., Lanaspa, M.A. and Johnson, R.J. (2020) Hyperosmolarity and increased serum sodium concentration are risks for developing hypertension regardless of salt intake: a five-year cohort study in Japan. *Nutrients* 12: 1422.

Perez-Pozo, S.E., Schold, J., Nakagawa, T., Sanchez-Lozada, L.G., Johnson, R.J. and Lillo, J.L. (2010) Excessive fructose intake induces the features of metabolic syndrome in healthy adult men: role of uric acid in the hypertensive response. *Int J Obes (Lond)* 34: 454–461.

Brymora, A., Flisiński, M., Johnson, R.J., Goszka, G., Stefańska, A. and Manitius, J. (2012) Low-fructose diet lowers blood pressure and inflammation in patients with chronic kidney disease. *Nephrol Dial Transplant* 27: 608–612.

Rodriguez-Iturbe, B., Pons, H. and Johnson, R.J. (2017) Role of the immune system in hypertension. *Physiol Rev* 97: 1127–1164.

Fatty Liver

Jensen, T., Abdelmalek, M.F., Sullivan, S., Nadeau, K.J., Green, M., Roncal, C., Nakagawa, T., Kuwabara, M., Sato, Y., Kang, D.H., Tolan, D.R., Sanchez-Lozada, L.G., Rosen, H.R., Lanaspa, M.A., Diehl, A.M. and Johnson, R.J. (2018) Fructose and sugar: A major mediator of non-alcoholic fatty liver disease. *J Hepatol* 68: 1063–1075.

Schwimmer, J.B., Ugalde-Nicalo, P., Welsh, J.A., Angeles, J.E., Cordero, M., Harlow, K.E., Alazraki, A., Durelle, J., Knight-Scott, J., Newton, K.P., Cleeton, R., Knott, C., Konomi, J., Middleton, M.S., Travers, C., Sirlin, C.B., Hernandez, A., Sekkarie, A., McCracken, C. and Vos, M.B. (2019) Effect of a low free sugar diet vs usual diet on nonalcoholic fatty liver disease in adolescent boys: a randomized clinical trial. *JAMA* 321: 256–265.

Ouyang, X., Cirillo, P., Sautin, Y., McCall, S., Bruchette, J.L., Diehl, A.M., Johnson, R.J. and Abdelmalek, M.F. (2008) Fructose consumption as a risk factor for non-alcoholic fatty liver disease. *J Hepatol* 48: 993–999.

Sánchez-Lozada, L.G., Mu, W., Roncal, C., Sautin, Y.Y., Abdelmalek, M., Reungjui, S., Le, M., Nakagawa, T., Lan, H.Y., Yu, X. and Johnson, R.J. (2010) Comparison of free fructose and glucose to sucrose in the ability to cause fatty liver. *Eur J Nutr* 49: 1–9.

Abdelmalek, M.F., Lazo, M., Horska, A., Bonekamp, S., Lipkin, E.W., Balasubramanyam, A., Bantle, J.P., Johnson, R.J., Diehl, A.M. and Clark, J.M. (2012) Higher dietary fructose is associated with impaired hepatic adenosine triphosphate homeostasis in obese individuals with type 2 diabetes. *Hepatology* 56: 952–960.

Maersk, M., Belza, A., Stodkilde-Jorgensen, H., Ringgaard, S., Chabanova, E., Thomsen, H., Pedersen, S.B., Astrup, A. and Richelsen, B. (2012) Sucrose-sweetened beverages increase fat storage in the liver, muscle, and visceral fat depot: a 6-mo randomized intervention study. *Am J Clin Nutr* 95: 283–289.

Chronic Kidney Disease

Gersch, M.S., Mu, W., Cirillo, P., Reungjui, S., Zhang, L., Roncal, C., Sautin, Y.Y., Johnson, R.J. and Nakagawa, T. (2007) Fructose, but not dextrose, accelerates the progression of chronic kidney disease. *Am J Physiol Renal Physiol* 293: F1256–1261.

Nakayama, T., Kosugi, T., Gersch, M., Connor, T., Sanchez-Lozada, L.G., Lanaspa, M.A., Roncal, C., Perez-Pozo, S.E., Johnson, R.J. and Nakagawa, T. (2010) Dietary fructose causes tubulointerstitial injury in the normal rat kidney. *Am J Physiol Renal Physiol* 298(3): F712–F720.

Cirillo, P., Gersch, M.S., Mu, W., Scherer, P.M., Kim, K.M., Gesualdo, L., Henderson, G.N., Johnson, R.J. and Sautin, Y.Y. (2009) Ketohexokinase-dependent metabolism of fructose induces proinflammatory mediators in proximal tubular cells. *J Am Soc Nephrol* 20(3): 545–553.

Sato, Y., Feig, D.I., Stack, A.G., Kang, D.H., Lanaspa, M.A., Ejaz, A.A., Sánchez-Lozada, L.G., Kuwabara, M., Borghi, C. and Johnson, R.J. (2019) The case for uric acid-lowering treatment in patients with hyperuricaemia and CKD. *Nat Rev Nephrol* 15(12): 767–775.

Badve, S.V., Pascoe, E.M., Tiku, A., Boudville, N., Brown, F.G., Cass, A., Clarke, P., Dalbeth, N., Day, R.O., de Zoysa, J.R., Douglas, B., Faull, R., Harris, D.C., Hawley, C.M., Jones, G.R.D., Kanellis, J., Palmer, S.C., Perkovic, V., Rangan, G.K., Reidlinger, D., Robison, L., Walker, R.J., Walters, G., Johnson, D.W. and CKD-FIX Study Investigators. (2020) Effects of allopurinol on the progression of chronic kidney disease. *N Engl J Med* 382: 2504–2513.

Doria, A., Galecki, A.T., Spino, C., et al. (2020) Serum urate lowering with allopurinol and kidney function in type 1 diabetes. *N Engl J Med* 382: 2493–2503.

Lanaspa, M.A., Ishimoto, T., Cicerchi, C., Tamura, Y., Roncal-Jimenez, C.A., Chen, W., Tanabe, K., Andres-Hernando, A., Orlicky, D.J., Finol, E., Inaba, S., Li, N., Rivard, C.J., Kosugi, T., Sanchez-Lozada, L.G., Petrash, J.M., Sautin, Y.Y., Ejaz, A.A., Kitagawa, W., Garcia, G.E., Bonthron, D.T., Asipu, A., Diggle, C.P., Rodriguez-Iturbe, B., Nakagawa, T. and Johnson, R.J. (2014) Endogenous fructose production and fructokinase activation mediate renal injury in diabetic nephropathy. *J Am Soc Nephrol* 25: 2526–2538.

Heart Disease

Yang, Q., Zhang, Z., Gregg, E.W., Flanders, W.D., Merritt, R. and Hu, F.B. (2014) Added sugar intake and cardiovascular diseases mortality among US adults. *JAMA Intern Med.* 174(4): 516–524.

Patetsios, P., Song, M., Shutze, W.P., Pappas, C., Rodino, W., Ramirez, J.A. and Panetta T.F. (2001) Identification of uric acid and xanthine oxidase in atherosclerotic plaque. *Am J Cardiol* 88: 188–191.

Cancer

Nakagawa, T., Lanaspa, M.A., Millan, I.S., Fini, M., Rivard, C.J., Sanchez-Lozada, L.G., Andres-Hernando, A., Tolan, D.R. and Johnson, R.J. (2020) Fructose contributes to the Warburg effect for cancer growth. *Cancer Metab* 8: 16.

Goncalves, M.D., Lu, C., Tutnauer, J., Hartman, T.E., Hwang, S.K., Murphy, C.J., Pauli, C., Morris, R., Taylor, S., Bosch, K., Yang, S., Wang, Y., Van Riper, J., Lekaye, H.C., Roper, J.,

Kim, Y., Chen, Q., Gross, S.S., Rhee, K.Y., Cantley, L.C. and Yun, J. (2019) High-fructose corn syrup enhances intestinal tumor growth in mice. *Science* 363: 1345–1349.

Park, T.J., Reznick, J., Peterson, B.L., Blass, G., Omerbasic, D., Bennett, N.C., Kuich, P., Zasada, C., Browe, B.M., Hamann, W., Applegate, D.T., Radke, M.H., Kosten, T., Lutermann, H., Gavaghan, V., Eigenbrod, O., Begay, V., Amoroso, V.G., Govind, V., Minshall, R.D., Smith, E.S.J., Larson, J., Gotthardt, M., Kempa, S. and Lewin, G.R. (2017) Fructose-driven glycolysis supports anoxia resistance in the naked mole-rat. *Science* 356: 307–311.

San Millán, I. and Brooks, G.A. (2017) Reexamining cancer metabolism: lactate production for carcinogenesis could be the purpose and explanation of the Warburg Effect. *Carcinogenesis* 38: 119–133.

Fini, M.A., Lanaspa, M.A., Gaucher, E.A., Boutwell, B., Nakagawa. T., Wright, R.M., Sanchez-Lozada, L.G., Andrews, P., Stenmark, K. and Johnson, R.J. (2021) Brief report: The uricase mutation in humans increases our risk for cancer growth. *Cancer Metab.* 15;9(1): 32.

Chapter 7: How the Survival Switch Affects Our Mind and Behavior

Alcohol

Avena, N.M., Rada, P. and Hoebel, B.G. (2008) Evidence for sugar addiction: behavioral and neurochemical effects of intermittent, excessive sugar intake. *Neurosci Biobehav Rev* 32: 20–39.

Lustig, R.H. (2013) Fructose: it's "alcohol without the buzz." *Adv Nutr* 4: 226–235.

Bouhlal, S., Farokhnia, M., Lee, M.R., Akhlaghi, F. and Leggio, L. (2018) Identifying and characterizing subpopulations of heavy alcohol drinkers via a sucrose preference test: a sweet road to a better phenotypic characterization? *Alcohol* 53: 560–569.

Fortuna, J.L. (2010) Sweet preference, sugar addiction and the familial history of alcohol dependence: shared neural pathways and genes. *J Psychoactive Drugs* 42: 147–151.

Andres-Hernando, A., Garcia, G.E., Orlicky, D.J., Loetz, E.C., Kumar, V., Effinger, D., Kuwabara, M., Bae, S.Y., Bell, R.L., Grahame, N.J., Kim, H., Dugar, S., Maffuid, P., Nakagawa, T., Wempe, M.F., Tolan, D.R., Bland, S.T., Johnson, R.J. and Lanaspa-Garcia, M.A. (2021) Alcohol preference and liver disease are dependent on sugar (fructose) metabolism. *Cell Metab* (submitted).

Wang, M., Chen, W.Y., Zhang, J., Gobejishvili, L., Barve, S.S., McClain, C.J. and Joshi-Barve, S. (2020) Elevated fructose and uric acid through aldose reductase contribute to experimental and human alcoholic liver disease. *Hepatology* 72: 1617–1637.

Barrio-Lopez, M.T., Bes-Rastrollo, M., Sayon-Orea, C., Garcia-Lopez, M., Fernandez-Montero, A., Gea, A. and Martinez-Gonzalez, M.A. (2013) Different types of alcoholic beverages and incidence of metabolic syndrome and its components in a Mediterranean cohort. *Clin Nutr* 32: 797–804.

Kotronen, A., Yki-Järvinen, H., Männistö, S., Saarikoski, L., Korpi-Hyövälti, E., Oksa, H., Saltevo, J., Saaristo, T., Sundvall, J., Tuomilehto, J. and Peltonen, M. (2010) Non-alcoholic and alcoholic fatty liver disease—two diseases of affluence associated with the metabolic syndrome and type 2 diabetes: the FIN-D2D survey. *BMC Public Health* 10: 237.

Shi, C., Wang, Y., Gao, J., Chen, S., Zhao, X., Cai, C., Guo, C. and Qiu, L. (2017) Inhibition of aldose reductase ameliorates alcoholic liver disease by activating AMPK and modulating oxidative stress and inflammatory cytokines. *Mol Med Rep* 16: 2767–2772.

Carn, D., Lanaspa, M., Benner, S., Andrews, P., Dudley, R., Andres-Hernando, A., Tolan, D.R. and Johnson, R.J. (2021) The role of thrifty genes in the origin of alcoholism: a narrative review and hypothesis. *Alcoholism: Clinical and Experimental Research* 45(8): 1519–1526.

Carrigan, M.A., Uryasev, O., Frye, C.B., Eckman, B.L., Myers, C.R., Hurley, T.D. and Benner, S.A. (2015) Hominids adapted to metabolize ethanol long before human-directed fermentation. *Proc Natl Acad Sci U S A* 112: 458–463.

Duncan, B.B., Chambless, L.E., Schmidt, M.I., Folsom, A.R., Szklo, M., Crouse, J.R., 3rd and Carpenter, M.A. (1995) Association of the waist-to-hip ratio is different with wine than with beer or hard liquor consumption. Atherosclerosis Risk in Communities Study Investigators. *Am J Epidemiol* 142: 1034–1038.

Fructose, Uric Acid, and Foraging

Johnson, R.J., Wilson, W.H., Bland, S.T. and Lanaspa, M.A. (2021) Fructose and uric acid as drivers of a hyperactive foraging response: A clue to behavioral disorders associated with impulsivity or mania? *Evolution and Human Behavior* 42: 194–203.

Luo, S., Monterosso, J.R., Sarpelleh, K. and Page, K.A. (2015) Differential effects of fructose versus glucose on brain and appetitive responses to food cues and decisions for food rewards. *Proc Natl Acad Sci U S A* 112: 6509–6514.

Purnell, J.Q., Klopfenstein, B.A., Stevens, A.A., Havel, P.J., Adams, S.H., Dunn, T.N., Krisky, C. and Rooney, W.D. (2011) Brain functional magnetic resonance imaging response to glucose and fructose infusions in humans. *Diabetes Obes Metab* 13: 229–234.

Sutin, A.R., Cutler, R.G., Camandola, S., Uda, M., Feldman, N.H., Cucca, F., Zonderman, A.B., Mattson, M.P., Ferrucci, L., Schlessinger, D. and Terracciano, A. (2014) Impulsivity is associated with uric acid: evidence from humans and mice. *Biol Psychiatry* 75: 31–37.

Cutler, R.G., Camandola, S., Feldman, N.H., Yoon, J.S., Haran, J.B., Arguelles, S. and Mattson, M.P. (2019) Uric acid enhances longevity and endurance and protects the brain against ischemia. *Neurobiol Aging* 75: 159–168.

Lane, M.D. and Cha, S.H. (2009) Effect of glucose and fructose on food intake via malonyl-CoA signaling in the brain. *Biochem Biophys Res Commun* 382: 1–5.

Barrera, C.M., Ruiz, Z.R. and Dunlap, W.P. (1988) Uric acid: a participating factor in the symptoms of hyperactivity. *Biol Psychiatry* 24: 344–347.

Lorenzi, T.M., Borba, D.L., Dutra, G. and Lara, D.R. (2010) Association of serum uric acid levels with emotional and affective temperaments. *J Affect Disord* 121: 161–164.

Robin, J.P., Boucontet, L., Chillet, P. and Groscolas, R. (1998) Behavioral changes in fasting emperor penguins: evidence for a "refeeding signal" linked to a metabolic shift. *Am J Physiol* 274(3): R746–753.

Hyperactivity and ADHD

Johnson, R.J., Gold, M.S., Johnson, D.R., Ishimoto, T., Lanaspa, M.A., Zahniser, N.R. and Avena, N.M. (2011) Attention-deficit/hyperactivity disorder: is it time to reappraise the role of sugar consumption? *Postgrad Med.* 123(5): 39–49.

Visser, S.N., Danielson, M.L., Bitsko, R.H., Holbrook, J.R., Kogan, M.D., Ghandour, R.M., Perou, R. and Blumberg, S.J. (2014) Trends in the parent-report of health care provider-diagnosed and medicated attention-deficit/hyperactivity disorder: United States, 2003–2011. *J Am Acad Child Adolesc Psychiatry* 53: 34–46 e32.

Hoerr, J., Fogel, J. and Van Voorhees, B. (2017) Ecological correlations of dietary food intake and mental health disorders. *J Epidemiol Glob Health* 7: 81–89.

Lien, L., Lien, N., Heyerdahl, S., Thoresen, M. and Bjertness, E. (2006) Consumption of soft drinks and hyperactivity, mental distress, and conduct problems among adolescents in Oslo, Norway. *Am J Public Health* 96: 1815–1820.

Barrera, C.M., Ruiz, Z.R. and Dunlap, W.P. (1988) Uric acid: a participating factor in the symptoms of hyperactivity. *Biol Psychiatry* 24: 344–347.

Van den Driessche, C., Chevrier, F., Cleeremans, A. and Sackur, J. (2019) Lower attentional skills predict increased exploratory foraging patterns. *Sci Rep* 9: 10948.

DiBattista, D. and Shepherd, M.L. (1993) Primary school teachers' beliefs and advice to parents concerning sugar consumption and activity in children. *Psychol Rep* 72(1): 47–55.

O'Reilly, G.A., Belcher, B.R., Davis, J.N., Martinez, L.T., Huh, J., Antunez-Castillo, L., Weigensberg, M., Goran, M.I. and Spruijt-Metz, D. (2015) Effects of high-sugar and high-fiber meals on physical activity behaviors in Latino and African American adolescents. *Obesity (Silver Spring)* 23: 1886–1894.

Wolraich, M.L., Lindgren, S.D., Stumbo, P.J., Stegink, L.D., Appelbaum, M.I. and Kiritsy, M.C. (1994) Effects of diets high in sucrose or aspartame on the behavior and cognitive performance of children. *N Engl J Med* 330: 301–307.

Franco-Perez, J., Manjarrez-Marmolejo, J., Ballesteros-Zebadua, P., Neri-Santos, A., Montes, S., Suarez-Rivera, N., Hernandez-Ceron, M. and Perez-Koldenkova, V. (2018) Chronic consumption of fructose induces behavioral alterations by increasing orexin and dopamine levels in the rat brain. *Nutrients* 10: 1722.

Hill, S.E., Prokosch, M.L., Morin, A. and Rodeheffer, C.D. (2014) The effect of non-caloric sweeteners on cognition, choice, and post-consumption satisfaction. *Appetite* 83: 82–88.

Ptacek, R., Kuzelova, H., Stefano, G.B., Raboch, J., Sadkova, T., Goetz, M. and Kream, R.M. (2014) Disruptive patterns of eating behaviors and associated lifestyles in males with ADHD. *Med Sci Monit* 20: 608–613.

Pagoto, S.L., Curtin, C., Lemon, S.C., Bandini, L.G., Schneider, K.L., Bodenlos, J.S. and Ma, Y. (2009) Association between adult attention deficit/hyperactivity disorder and obesity in the US population. *Obesity (Silver Spring)* 17: 539–544.

Agranat-Meged, A.N., Deitcher, C., Goldzweig, G., Leibenson, L., Stein, M. and Galili-Weisstub, E. (2005) Childhood obesity and attention deficit/hyperactivity disorder: a newly described comorbidity in obese hospitalized children. *Int J Eat Disord* 37: 357–359.

Altfas, J.R. (2002) Prevalence of attention deficit/hyperactivity disorder among adults in obesity treatment. *BMC Psychiatry* 2: 9.

Bipolar Disorder and Depression

Blader, J.C. and Carlson, G.A. (2007) Increased rates of bipolar disorder diagnoses among U.S. child, adolescent, and adult inpatients, 1996–2004. *Biol Psychiatry* 62: 107–114.

Kessing, L.V., Vradi, E. and Andersen, P.K. (2014) Are rates of pediatric bipolar disorder increasing? Results from a nationwide register study. *Int J Bipolar Disord* 2: 10.

Elmslie, J.L., Mann, J.I., Silverstone, J.T., Williams, S.M. and Romans, S.E. (2001) Determinants of overweight and obesity in patients with bipolar disorder. *J Clin Psychiatry* 62: 486–491; quiz 492–483.

Kesebir, S., Tatlıdil Yaylacı, E., Süner. O. and Gültekin, B.K. (2014) Uric acid levels may be a biological marker for the differentiation of unipolar and bipolar disorder: the role of affective temperament. *J Affect Disord* 165: 131–134.

Shorter, E. (2009) The history of lithium therapy. *Bipolar Disord* 11 Suppl 2: 4–9.

Akhondzadeh, S., Milajerdi, M.R., Amini, H. and Tehrani-Doost, M. (2006) Allopurinol as an adjunct to lithium and haloperidol for treatment of patients with acute mania: a double-blind, randomized, placebo-controlled trial. *Bipolar Disord* 8: 485–489.

Fan, A., Berg, A., Bresee, C., Glassman, L.H. and Rapaport, M.H. (2012) Allopurinol augmentation in the outpatient treatment of bipolar mania: a pilot study. *Bipolar Disord* 14: 206–210.

Jahangard, L., Soroush, S., Haghighi, M., Ghaleiha, A., Bajoghli, H., Holsboer-Trachsler, E. and Brand, S. (2014) In a double-blind, randomized and placebo-controlled trial, adjuvant allopurinol improved symptoms of mania in in-patients suffering from bipolar disorder. *Eur Neuropsychopharmacol* 24: 1210–1221.

Machado-Vieira, R., Soares, J.C., Lara, D.R., Luckenbaugh, D.A., Busnello, J.V., Marca, G., Cunha, A., Souza, D.O., Zarate, C.A., Jr. and Kapczinski, F. (2008) A double-blind, randomized, placebo-controlled 4-week study on the efficacy and safety of the purinergic agents allopurinol and dipyridamole adjunctive to lithium in acute bipolar mania. *J Clin Psychiatry* 69: 1237–1245.

Regenold, W.T., Hisley, K.C., Phatak, P., Marano, C.M., Obuchowski, A., Lefkowitz, D.M., Sassan, A., Ohri, S., Phillips, T.L., Dosanjh, N., Conley, R.R. and Gullapalli, R. (2008) Relationship of cerebrospinal fluid glucose metabolites to MRI deep white matter hyperintensities and treatment resistance in bipolar disorder patients. *Bipolar Disord* 10: 753–764.

Regenold, W.T., Phatak, P., Kling, M.A. and Hauser, P. (2004) Post-mortem evidence from human brain tissue of disturbed glucose metabolism in mood and psychotic disorders. *Mol Psychiatry* 9: 731–733.

Knuppel, A., Shipley, M.J., Llewellyn, C.H. and Brunner, E.J. (2017) Sugar intake from sweet food and beverages, common mental disorder and depression: prospective findings from the Whitehall II study. *Sci Rep* 7: 6287.

Westover, A.N. and Marangell, L.B. (2002) A cross-national relationship between sugar consumption and major depression? *Depress Anxiety* 16: 118–120.

Sanchez-Lozada, L.G., Andres-Hernando, A., Garcia-Arroyo, F.E., Cicerchi, C., Li, N., Kuwabara, M., Roncal-Jimenez, C.A., Johnson, R.J. and Lanaspa, M.A. (2019) Uric acid activates aldose reductase and the polyol pathway for endogenous fructose and fat production causing development of fatty liver in rats. *J Biol Chem* 294: 4272–4281.

Aggression

Solnick, S.J. and Hemenway, D. (2012) The "Twinkie Defense": the relationship between carbonated non-diet soft drinks and violence perpetration among Boston high school students. *Inj Prev* 18: 259–263.

Solnick, S.J. and Hemenway, D. (2014) Soft drinks, aggression and suicidal behaviour in US high school students. *Int J Inj Contr Saf Promot* 21: 266–273.

Moore, S.C., Carter, L.M. and van Goozen, S. (2009) Confectionery consumption in childhood and adult violence. *Br J Psychiatry* 195: 366–367.

Spitz, R.T., Hillbrand, M. and Foster, H.G. (1995) Uric acid levels and severity of aggression. *Psychol Rep* 76: 130.

Grover, C.D., Kay, A.D., Monson, J.A., Marsh, T.C. and Holway, D.A. (2007) Linking nutrition and behavioural dominance: carbohydrate scarcity limits aggression and activity in Argentine ants. *Proc Biol Sci* 274: 2951–2957.

Carroll, C.R. and Janzen, D.H. (1973) Ecology of foraging by ants. *Annual Review of Ecology and Systematics* 4: 231–257.

Alzheimer's Disease

Johnson, R.J., Gomez-Pinilla, F., Nagel, M., Nakagawa, T., Rodriguez-Iturbe, B., Sanchez-Lozada, L.G., Tolan, D.R. and Lanaspa, M.A. (2020) Cerebral fructose metabolism as a potential mechanism driving Alzheimer's disease. *Front Aging Neurosci* 12: 560865.

Neth, B.J. and Craft, S. (2017) Insulin resistance and Alzheimer's disease: bioenergetic linkages. *Front Aging Neurosci* 9: 345.

Cenini, G. and Voos, W. (2019) Mitochondria as potential targets in Alzheimer Disease therapy: an update. *Front Pharmacol* 10: 902.

Kendig, M.D., Boakes, R.A., Rooney, K.B. and Corbit, L.H. (2013) Chronic restricted access to 10% sucrose solution in adolescent and young adult rats impairs spatial memory and alters sensitivity to outcome devaluation. *Physiol Behav* 120: 164–172.

Agrawal, R., Noble, E., Vergnes, L., Ying, Z., Reue, K. and Gomez-Pinilla, F. (2016) Dietary fructose aggravates the pathobiology of traumatic brain injury by influencing energy homeostasis and plasticity. *J Cereb Blood Flow Metab* 36: 941–953.

Xu, J., Begley, P., Church, S.J., Patassini, S., McHarg, S., Kureishy, N., Hollywood, K.A., Waldvogel, H.J., Liu, H., Zhang, S., Lin, W., Herholz, K., Turner, C., Synek, B.J., Curtis, M.A., Rivers-Auty, J., Lawrence, C.B., Kellett, K.A., Hooper, N.M., Vardy, E.R., Wu, D., Unwin, R.D., Faull, R.L., Dowsey, A.W. and Cooper, G.J. (2016) Elevation of brain glucose and polyol-pathway intermediates with accompanying brain-copper deficiency in patients with Alzheimer's disease: metabolic basis for dementia. *Sci Rep* 6: 27524.

Sims, B., Powers, R.E., Sabina, R.L. and Theibert, A.B. (1998) Elevated adenosine monophosphate deaminase activity in Alzheimer's disease brain. *Neurobiol Aging* 19: 385–391.

Hoyer, S. (1994) Possible role of ammonia in the brain in dementia of Alzheimer type. *Adv Exp Med Biol* 368: 197–205.

Roberts, R.O., Roberts, L.A., Geda, Y.E., Cha, R.H., Pankratz, V.S., O'Connor, H.M., Knopman, D.S. and Petersen, R.C. (2012) Relative intake of macronutrients impacts risk of mild cognitive impairment or dementia. *J Alzheimers Dis* 32: 329–339.

Ge, Q., Wang, Z., Wu, Y., Huo, Q., Qian, Z., Tian, Z., Ren, W., Zhang, X. and Han, J. (2017) High salt diet impairs memory-related synaptic plasticity via increased oxidative stress and suppressed synaptic protein expression. *Mol Nutr Food Res* 61(10): 1700134.

Pase, M.P., Himali, J.J., Jacques, P.F., DeCarli, C., Satizabal, C.L., Aparicio, H., Vasan, R.S., Beiser, A.S. and Seshadri, S. (2017) Sugary beverage intake and preclinical Alzheimer's disease in the community. *Alzheimers Dement* 13: 955–964.

Burrows, T., Goldman, S., Olson, R.K., Byrne, B. and Coventry, W.L. (2017) Associations between selected dietary behaviours and academic achievement: A study of Australian school aged children. *Appetite* 116: 372–380.

Cao, D., Lu, H., Lewis, T.L. and Li, L. (2007) Intake of sucrose-sweetened water induces insulin resistance and exacerbates memory deficits and amyloidosis in a transgenic mouse model of Alzheimer disease. *J Biol Chem* 282: 36275–36282.

Simopoulos, A.P. (2013) Dietary omega-3 fatty acid deficiency and high fructose intake in the development of metabolic syndrome, brain metabolic abnormalities, and non-alcoholic fatty liver disease. *Nutrients* 5: 2901–2923.

Singh, J.A. and Cleveland, J.D. (2018) Comparative effectiveness of allopurinol versus febuxostat for preventing incident dementia in older adults: a propensity-matched analysis. *Arthritis Res Ther* 20: 167.

Schretlen, D.J., Inscore, A.B., Jinnah, H.A., Rao, V., Gordon, B. and Pearlson, G.D. (2007) Serum uric acid and cognitive function in community-dwelling older adults. *Neuropsychology* 21: 136–140.

The Uric Acid Paradox

Orowan, E. (1955) The origin of man. *Nature* 175: 683–684.

Kasl, S.V. (1974) Are there any promising biochemical correlates of achievement behavior and motivation? The evidence for serum uric acid and serum cholesterol. *Review of Educational Research* 44: 447–462.

Brooks, G.W. and Mueller, E. (1966) Serum urate concentrations among university professors; relation to drive, achievement, and leadership. *JAMA* 195: 415–418.

PART III: OUTFOXING NATURE

Chapter 8: Understanding Sugar in Our Diet

Current Sugar Intake and Recommendations

Ng, S.W., Slining, M.M. and Popkin, B.M. (2012) Use of caloric and noncaloric sweeteners in US consumer packaged foods, 2005–2009. *J Acad Nutr Diet* 112: 1828–1834.

Special Issue: U.S. beverage results for 2011. (2012) *Beverage Digest* 61: 2.

World Health Organization. (2015). Guideline: Sugars intake for adults and children. Geneva, Switzerland: World Health Organization: 1–59.

Johnson, R.K., Appel, L.J., Brands, M., Howard, B.V., Lefevre, M., Lustig, R.H., Sacks, F., Steffen, L.M. and Wylie-Rosett, J. (2009) Dietary sugars intake and cardiovascular health: a scientific statement from the American Heart Association. *Circulation* 120: 1011–1020.

Fruits and Sugar

Jang, C., Hui, S., Lu, W., Cowan, A.J., Morscher, R.J., Lee, G., Liu, W., Tesz, G.J., Birnbaum, M.J. and Rabinowitz, J.D. (2018) The small intestine converts dietary fructose into glucose and organic acids. *Cell Metab* 27: 351–361.

Jang, C., Wada, S., Yang, S., Gosis, B., Zeng, X., Zhang, Z., Shen, Y., Lee, G., Arany, Z. and Rabinowitz, J.D. (2020) The small intestine shields the liver from fructose-induced steatosis. *Nat Metab* 2: 586–593.

Andres-Hernando, A., Orlicky, D.J., Kuwabara, M., Ishimoto, T., Nakagawa, T., Johnson, R.J. and Lanaspa, M.A. (2020) Deletion of fructokinase in the liver or in the intestine reveals differential effects on sugar-induced metabolic dysfunction. *Cell Metab* 32(1): 117–127.

García-Arroyo, F.E., Gonzaga-Sánchez, G., Tapia, E., Muñoz-Jiménez, I., Manterola-Romero, L., Osorio-Alonso, H., Arellano-Buendía, A.S., Pedraza-Chaverri, J., Roncal-Jiménez, C.A., Lanaspa, M.A., Johnson, R.J. and Sánchez-Lozada, L.G. (2021) Osthol ameliorates kidney damage and metabolic syndrome induced by a high-fat/high-sugar diet. *Int J Mol Sci.* 22: 2431.

Zhang, J., Zhao, L., Cheng, Q., Ji, B., Yang, M., Sanidad, K.Z., Wang, C. and Zhou, F. (2018) Structurally different flavonoid subclasses attenuate high-fat and high-fructose diet induced metabolic syndrome in rats. *J Agric Food Chem* 66(46): 12412–12420.

Reungjui, S., Roncal, C.A., Mu, W., Srinivas, T.R., Sirivongs, D., Johnson, R.J., Nakagawa, T. (2007) Thiazide diuretics exacerbate fructose-induced metabolic syndrome. *J Am Soc Nephrol* 18: 2724–2731.

Madero, M., Arriaga, J.C., Jalal, D., Rivard, C., McFann, K., Perez-Mendez, O., Vazquez, A., Ruiz, A., Lanaspa, M.A., Jimenez, C.R., Johnson, R.J. and Lozada, L.G. (2011) The effect of two energy-restricted diets, a low-fructose diet versus a moderate natural fructose diet, on weight loss and metabolic syndrome parameters: a randomized controlled trial. *Metabolism* 60: 1551–1559.

American Academy of Pediatrics. (2001) The use and misuse of fruit juice in pediatrics. *Pediatrics* 107: 1210–1213.

Johnson, R.J. and Gower, T. (2008). *The Sugar Fix. The High-Fructose Fallout That Is Making You Fat and Sick*. New York, Rodale.

Sugary Drinks Versus Sugary Foods

Sundborn, G., Thornley, S., Merriman, T.R., Lang, B., King, C., Lanaspa, M.A. and Johnson, R.J. (2019) Are liquid sugars different from solid sugar in their ability to cause metabolic syndrome? *Obesity (Silver Spring)* 27: 879–887.

Togo, J., Hu, S., Li, M., Niu, C. and Speakman, J.R. (2019) Impact of dietary sucrose on adiposity and glucose homeostasis in C57BL/6J mice depends on mode of ingestion: liquid or solid. *Mol Metab* 27: 22–32.

Kanbay, M., Guler, G., Ertuglu, L.A., Dagel, T., Afsar, B., Incir, S., Baygul, A., Covic, A., Andres-Hernando, A., Sanchez-Lozada, L.G., Lanaspa, M.A. and Johnson, R.J. (2021) The speed of ingestion of a sugary beverage has an effect on the acute metabolic response to fructose. *Nutrients* 13(6): 1916.

DiMeglio, D.P. and Mattes, R.D. (2000) Liquid versus solid carbohydrate: effects on food intake and body weight. *Int J Obes Relat Metab Disord* 24: 794–800.

Fructose Regulates Its Uptake and Metabolism

Roncal-Jimenez, C.A., Lanaspa, M.A., Rivard, C.J., Nakagawa, T., Sanchez-Lozada, L.G., Jalal, D., Andres-Hernando, A., Tanabe, K., Madero, M., Li, N., Cicerchi, C., Mc Fann, K., Sautin, Y.Y. and Johnson, R.J. (2011) Sucrose induces fatty liver and pancreatic inflammation in male breeder rats independent of excess energy intake. *Metabolism* 60: 1259–1270.

Lanaspa, M.A., Sanchez-Lozada, L.G., Cicerchi, C., Li, N., Roncal-Jimenez, C.A., Ishimoto, T., Le, M., Garcia, G.E., Thomas, J.B., Rivard, C.J., Andres-Hernando, A., Hunter, B., Schreiner, G., Rodriguez-Iturbe, B., Sautin, Y.Y. and Johnson, R.J. (2012) Uric acid stimulates fructokinase and accelerates fructose metabolism in the development of fatty liver. *PLoS One.* 7(10): e47948.

Sanchez-Lozada, L.G., Andres-Hernando, A., Garcia-Arroyo, F.E., Cicerchi, C., Li, N., Kuwabara, M., Roncal-Jimenez, C.A., Johnson, R.J. and Lanaspa, M.A. (2019) Uric acid activates aldose reductase and the polyol pathway for endogenous fructose and fat production causing development of fatty liver in rats. *J Biol Chem* 294: 4272–4281.

Burant, C.F. and Saxena, M. (1994) Rapid reversible substrate regulation of fructose transporter expression in rat small intestine and kidney. *Am J Physiol* 267: G71–79.

Garcia-Arroyo, F.E., Monroy-Sanchez, F., Munoz-Jimenez, I., Gonzaga, G., Andres-Hernando, A., Zazueta, C., Juarez-Rojas, J.G., Lanaspa, M.A., Johnson, R.J. and Sanchez-Lozada, L.G. (2019) Allopurinol prevents the lipogenic response induced by an acute oral fructose challenge in short-term fructose fed rats. *Biomolecules* 9: 601.

Sullivan, J.S., Le, M.T., Pan, Z., Rivard, C., Love-Osborne, K., Robbins, K., Johnson, R.J., Sokol, R.J. and Sundaram, S.S. (2015) Oral fructose absorption in obese children with non-alcoholic fatty liver disease. *Pediatr Obes* 10: 188–195.

Artificial Sugars

Choudhary, A.K. and Lee, Y.Y. (2018) Neurophysiological symptoms and aspartame: What is the connection? *Nutr Neurosci* 21: 306–316.

Abdel-Salam, O.M., Salem, N.A., El-Shamarka, M.E., Hussein, J.S., Ahmed, N.A. and El-Nagar, M.E. (2012) Studies on the effects of aspartame on memory and oxidative stress in brain of mice. *Eur Rev Med Pharmacol Sci* 16: 2092–2101.

Sylvetsky, A.C., Figueroa, J., Zimmerman, T., Swithers, S.E. and Welsh, J.A. (2019) Consumption of low-calorie sweetened beverages is associated with higher total energy and sugar intake among children, NHANES 2011–2016. *Pediatr Obes* 14: e12535.

Hill, S.E., Prokosch, M.L., Morin, A. and Rodeheffer, C.D. (2014) The effect of non-caloric sweeteners on cognition, choice, and post-consumption satisfaction. *Appetite* 83: 82–88.

Andres-Hernando, A., Kuwabara, M., Orlicky, D.J., Vandenbeuch, A., Cicerchi, C., Kinnamon, S.C., Finger, T.E., Johnson, R.J. and Lanaspa, M.A. (2020) Sugar causes obesity and metabolic syndrome in mice independently of sweet taste. *Am J Physiol Endocrinol Metab.* 319: E276–E290.

Suez, J., Korem, T., Zeevi, D., Zilberman-Schapira, G., Thaiss, C.A., Maza, O., Israeli, D., Zmora, N., Gilad, S., Weinberger, A., Kuperman, Y., Harmelin, A., Kolodkin-Gal, I., Shapiro, H., Halpern, Z., Segal, E. and Elinav, E. (2014) Artificial sweeteners induce glucose intolerance by altering the gut microbiota. *Nature* 514: 181–186.

Johnson, R.J., Rivard, C., Lanaspa, M.A., Otabachian-Smith, S., Ishimoto, T., Cicerchi, C., Cheeke, P.R., Macintosh, B. and Hess, T. (2013) Fructokinase, fructans, intestinal permeability, and metabolic syndrome: an equine connection? *J Equine Vet Science* 33: 120–126.

Sports Drinks

Cade, J.R., Free, H.J., De Quesada, A.M., Shires, D.L. and Roby, L. (1971) Changes in body fluid composition and volume during vigorous exercise by athletes. *J Sports Med Phys Fitness* 11: 172–178.

Johnson, R.J. and Murray, R. (2010) Fructose, exercise, and health. *Curr Sports Med Rep* 9: 253–258.

Dougherty, K.A., Baker, L.B., Chow, M. and Kenney, W.L. (2006) Two percent dehydration impairs and six percent carbohydrate drink improves boys basketball skills. *Med Sci Sports Exerc* 38: 1650–1658.

Glucose and Performance

Owen, L., Scholey, A.B., Finnegan, Y., Hu, H. and Sunram-Lea, S.I. (2012) The effect of glucose dose and fasting interval on cognitive function: a double-blind, placebo-controlled, six-way crossover study. *Psychopharmacology (Berl)* 220: 577–589.

Rampersaud, G.C., Pereira, M.A., Girard, B.L., Adams, J. and Metzl, J.D. (2005) Breakfast habits, nutritional status, body weight, and academic performance in children and adolescents. *J Am Diet Assoc* 105: 743–760; quiz 761–762.

Cooper, S.B., Bandelow, S., Nute, M.L., Morris, J.G. and Nevill, M.E. (2012) Breakfast glycaemic index and cognitive function in adolescent school children. *Br J Nutr* 107: 1823–1832.

Benton, D. and Parker, P.Y. (1998) Breakfast, blood glucose, and cognition. *Am J Clin Nutr.* 67: 772S–778S.

Sugar Resistance

Pontzer, H. (2017) The exercise paradox. *Sci Am* 316: 26–31.

Marlowe, F.W., Berbesque, J.C., Wood, B., Crittenden, A., Porter, C. and Mabulla, A. (2014) Honey, Hadza, hunter-gatherers, and human evolution. *J Hum Evol* 71: 119–128.

Crittenden, A.N., Sorrentino, J., Moonie, S.A., Peterson, M., Mabulla, A. and Ungar, P.S. (2017) Oral health in transition: The Hadza foragers of Tanzania. *PLoS One* 12: e0172197.

Leonidas, J.C. (1965) Essential fructosuria. *N Y State J Med* 65: 2257–2259.

Bayard, V., Chamorro, F., Motta, J. and Hollenberg, N.K. (2007) Does flavanol intake influence mortality from nitric oxide-dependent processes? Ischemic heart disease, stroke, diabetes mellitus, and cancer in Panama. *Int J Med Sci* 4: 53–58.

Hollenberg, N.K., Rivera, A., Meinking, T., Martinez, G., McCullough, M., Passan, D., Preston, M., Taplin, D. and Vicaria-Clement, M. (1999) Age, renal perfusion and function in island-dwelling indigenous Kuna Amerinds of Panama. *Nephron* 82: 131–138.

Gutiérrez-Salmeán, G., Meaney, E., Lanaspa, M.A., Cicerchi, C., Johnson, R.J., Dugar, S., Taub, P., Ramírez-Sánchez, I., Villarreal, F., Schreiner, G. and Ceballos, G. (2016) A randomized, placebo-controlled, double-blind study on the effects of (-)-epicatechin on the triglyceride/HDLc ratio and cardiometabolic profile of subjects with hypertriglyceridemia: Unique in vitro effects. *Int J Cardiol* 223: 500–506.

Chapter 9: The Optimal Diet for Blocking the Fat Switch

Glycemic Index and General Nutrition

Atkinson, F.S., Foster-Powell, K. and Brand-Miller, J.C. (2008) International tables of glycemic index and glycemic load values. *Diabetes Care* 31: 2281–2283.

Foster-Powell, K., Holt, S.H. and Brand-Miller, J.C. (2002) International table of glycemic index and glycemic load values. *Am J Clin Nutr* 76: 5–56.

Mozaffarian, D., Hao, T., Rimm, E.B., Willett, W.C. and Hu, F.B. (2011) Changes in diet and lifestyle and long-term weight gain in women and men. *N Engl J Med* 364: 2392–2404.

Bendsen, N.T., Christensen, R., Bartels, E.M. and Astrup, A. (2011) Consumption of industrial and ruminant trans fatty acids and risk of coronary heart disease: a systematic review and meta-analysis of cohort studies. *Eur J Clin Nutr* 65: 773–783.

Shapiro, A., Tümer, N., Gao, Y., Cheng, K.Y. and Scarpace, P.J. (2011) Prevention and reversal of diet-induced leptin resistance with a sugar-free diet despite high fat content. *Br J Nutr* 106(3): 390–397.

Simopoulos, A.P. (2016) An increase in the omega-6/omega-3 fatty acid ratio increases the risk for obesity. *Nutrients* 8: 128.

Infante, J.P., Kirwan, R.C. and Brenna, J.T. (2001) High levels of docosahexaenoic acid (22:6n-3)-containing phospholipids in high-frequency contraction muscles of hummingbirds and rattlesnakes. *Comp Biochem Physiol B Biochem Mol Biol* 130: 291–298.

Schwingshackl, L., Hoffmann, G., Schwedhelm, C., Kalle-Uhlmann, T., Missbach, B., Knuppel, S. and Boeing, H. (2016) Consumption of dairy products in relation to changes in anthropometric variables in adult populations: a systematic review and meta-analysis of cohort studies. *PLoS One* 11: e0157461.

Thorning, T.K., Raben, A., Tholstrup, T., Soedamah-Muthu, S.S., Givens, I. and Astrup, A. (2016) Milk and dairy products: good or bad for human health? An assessment of the totality of scientific evidence. *Food Nutr Res* 60: 32527.

Wang, Y. and Beydoun, M.A. (2009) Meat consumption is associated with obesity and central obesity among US adults. *Int J Obes (Lond)* 33: 621–628.

Diet Studies

Andrews, P. and Johnson, R.J. (2020) Evolutionary basis for the human diet: consequences for human health. *J Intern Med* 287: 226–237.

Mozaffarian, D. (2016) Dietary and policy priorities for cardiovascular disease, diabetes, and obesity: a comprehensive review. *Circulation* 133: 187–225.

Ballard, K.D., Quann, E.E., Kupchak, B.R., Volk, B.M., Kawiecki, D.M., Fernandez, M.L., Seip, R.L., Maresh, C.M., Kraemer, W.J. and Volek, J.S. (2013) Dietary carbohydrate restriction improves insulin sensitivity, blood pressure, microvascular function, and cellular adhesion markers in individuals taking statins. *Nutr Res.* 33: 905–912.

Hyde, P.N., Sapper, T.N., Crabtree, C.D., LaFountain, R.A., Bowling, M.L., Buga, A., Fell, B., McSwiney, F.T., Dickerson, R.M., Miller, V.J., Scandling, D., Simonetti, O.P., Phinney, S.D., Kraemer, W.J., King, S.A., Krauss, R.M. and Volek, J.S. (2019) Dietary carbohydrate restriction improves metabolic syndrome independent of weight loss. *JCI Insight* 4: e128308.

Foster, G.D., Wyatt, H.R., Hill, J.O., Makris, A.P., Rosenbaum, D.L., Brill, C., Stein, R.I., Mohammed, B.S., Miller, B., Rader, D.J., Zemel, B., Wadden, T.A., Tenhave, T., Newcomb, C.W. and Klein, S. (2010) Weight and metabolic outcomes after 2 years on a low-carbohydrate versus low-fat diet: a randomized trial. *Ann Intern Med* 153: 147–157.

Samaha, F.F., Iqbal, N., Seshadri, P., Chicano, K.L., Daily, D.A., McGrory, J., Williams, T., Williams, M., Gracely, E.J. and Stern, L. (2003) A low-carbohydrate as compared with a low-fat diet in severe obesity. *N Engl J Med* 348: 2074–2081.

Mellberg, C., Sandberg, S., Ryberg, M., Eriksson, M., Brage, S., Larsson, C., Olsson, T. and Lindahl, B. (2014) Long-term effects of a Palaeolithic-type diet in obese postmenopausal women: a 2-year randomized trial. *Eur J Clin Nutr* 68: 350–357.

Sacks, F.M., Bray, G.A., Carey, V.J., Smith, S.R., Ryan, D.H., Anton, S.D., McManus, K., Champagne, C.M., Bishop, L.M., Laranjo, N., Leboff, M.S., Rood, J.C., de Jonge, L., Greenway, F.L., Loria, C.M., Obarzanek, E. and Williamson, D.A. (2009) Comparison of weight-loss diets with different compositions of fat, protein, and carbohydrates. *N Engl J Med* 360: 859–873.

Trichopoulou, A., Costacou, T., Bamia, C. and Trichopoulos, D. (2003) Adherence to a Mediterranean diet and survival in a Greek population. *N Engl J Med* 348: 2599–2608.

Mazidi, M., Katsiki, N., Mikhailidis, D.P., Sattar, N. and Banach, M. (2019) Lower carbohydrate diets and all-cause and cause-specific mortality: a population-based cohort study and pooling of prospective studies. *Eur Heart J* 40: 2870–2879.

Jospe, M.R., Roy, M., Brown, R.C., Haszard, J.J., Meredith-Jones, K., Fangupo, L.J., Osborne, H., Fleming, E.A. and Taylor, R.W. (2020) Intermittent fasting, Paleolithic, or Mediterranean diets in the real world: exploratory secondary analyses of a weight-loss trial that included choice of diet and exercise. *Am J Clin Nutr* 111: 503–514.

Volek, J.S., Phinney, S.D., Krauss, R.M., Johnson, R.J., Saslow, L.R., Gower, B., Yandy, W.W., King, J., Hecht, F.M., Teicholz, N., Bistrian, B.R., Hamdy, O. (2021) Alternative dietary patterns for Americans: Low-carbohydrate diet. *Nutrients* 13: 3299.

Sleep

Chaput, J.P., Tremblay, M.S., Katzmarzyk, P.T., Fogelholm, M., Hu, G., Maher, C., Maia, J., Olds, T., Onywera, V., Sarmiento, O.L., Standage, M., Tudor-Locke, C., Sampasa-Kanyinga, H. and Group, I.R. (2018) Sleep patterns and sugar-sweetened beverage consumption among children from around the world. *Public Health Nutr* 21: 2385–2393.

Markwald, R.R., Melanson, E.L., Smith, M.R., Higgins, J., Perreault, L., Eckel, R.H. and Wright, K.P., Jr. (2013) Impact of insufficient sleep on total daily energy expenditure, food intake, and weight gain. *Proc Natl Acad Sci U S A* 110: 5695–5700.

Chen, X., Beydoun, M.A. and Wang, Y. (2008) Is sleep duration associated with childhood obesity? A systematic review and meta-analysis. *Obesity (Silver Spring)* 16: 265–274.

Potential Benefit of Continuous Glucose Monitoring

Zeevi, D., Korem, T., Zmora, N., Israeli, D., Rothschild, D., Weinberger, A., Ben-Yacov, O., Lador, D., Avnit-Sagi, T., Lotan-Pompan, M., Suez, J., Mahdi, J.A., Matot, E., Malka, G., Kosower, N., Rein, M., Zilberman-Schapira, G., Dohnalová, L., Pevsner-Fischer, M., Bikovsky, R., Halpern, Z., Elinav, E. and Segal, E. (2015) Personalized nutrition by prediction of glycemic responses. *Cell* 163: 1079–1094.

Hall, H., Perelman, D., Breschi, A., Limcaoco, P., Kellogg, R., McLaughlin, T. and Snyder, M. (2018) Glucotypes reveal new patterns of glucose dysregulation. *PLoS Biol.* 16: e2005143.

Hydration

Stookey, J.J. (2016) Negative, null and beneficial effects of drinking water on energy intake, energy expenditure, fat oxidation and weight change in randomized trials: a qualitative review. *Nutrients* 8: 19.

Stookey, J.D., Kavouras, S., Suh, H. and Lang, F. (2020) Underhydration is associated with obesity, chronic diseases, and death within 3 to 6 years in the U.S. population aged 51–70 years. *Nutrients* 12(4): 905.

Stookey, J.D. (2017) Under what conditions do water-intervention studies significantly improve child body weight? *Ann Nutr Metab* 70 Suppl 1: 62–67.

Lowering Uric Acid

Ejaz, A.A., Nakagawa, T., Kanbay, M., Kuwabara, M., Kumar, A., Garcia Arroyo, F.E., Roncal-Jimenez, C., Sasai, F., Kang, D.H., Jensen, T., Hernando, A.A., Rodriguez-Iturbe, B., Garcia, G., Tolan, D.R., Sanchez-Lozada, L.G., Lanaspa, M.A. and Johnson, R.J. (2020) Hyperuricemia in kidney disease: a major risk factor for cardiovascular events, vascular calcification, and renal damage. *Semin Nephrol* 40: 574–585.

Piani, F., Sasai F, Bjornstad, P., Borghi, C., Yoshimura, A., Sanchez-Lozada, L.G., Roncal-Jimenez, C., Garcia, G.E., Hernando, A.A., Fuentes, G.C., Rodriguez-Iturbe, B., Lanaspa, M.A., Johnson, R.J. (2021) Hyperuricemia and chronic kidney disease: to treat or not to treat. *J Bras Nefrol* S0101-28002021005026301.

Johnson, R.J., Bakris, G.L., Borghi, C., Chonchol, M.B., Feldman, D., Lanaspa, M.A., Merriman, T.R., Moe, O.W., Mount, D.B., Sanchez Lozada, L.G., Stahl, E., Weiner, D.E.

and Chertow, G.M. (2018) Hyperuricemia, acute and chronic kidney disease, hypertension, and cardiovascular disease: report of a scientific workshop organized by the National Kidney Foundation. *Am J Kidney Dis* 71: 851–865.

Chapter 10: Restoring Your Original Weight and Improving Your Healthspan

Gait Test

Hills, A.P. and Parker, A.W. (1991) Gait characteristics of obese children. *Arch Phys Med Rehabil* 72: 403–407.

Santanasto, A.J., Coen, P.M., Glynn, N.W., Conley, K.E., Jubrias, S.A., Amati, F., Strotmeyer, E.S., Boudreau, R.M., Goodpaster, B.H. and Newman, A.B. (2016) The relationship between mitochondrial function and walking performance in older adults with a wide range of physical function. *Exp Gerontol* 81: 1–7.

Luk, T.H., Dai, Y.L., Siu, C.W., Yiu, K.H., Li, S.W., Fong, B., Wong, W.K., Tam, S. and Tse, H.F. (2012) Association of lower habitual physical activity level with mitochondrial and endothelial dysfunction in patients with stable coronary artery disease. *Circ J* 76: 2572–2578.

Apabhai, S., Gorman, G.S., Sutton, L., Elson, J.L., Plotz, T., Turnbull, D.M. and Trenell, M.I. (2011) Habitual physical activity in mitochondrial disease. *PLoS One* 6: e22294.

Coen, P.M., Jubrias, S.A., Distefano, G., et al. (2013) Skeletal muscle mitochondrial energetics are associated with maximal aerobic capacity and walking speed in older adults. *J Gerontol A Biol Sci Med Sci* 68: 447–455.

Jerome, G.J., Ko, S.U., Chiles Shaffer, N.S., Studenski, S.A., Ferrucci, L. and Simonsick, E.M. (2016) Cross-sectional and longitudinal associations between adiposity and walking endurance in adults age 60–79. *J Gerontol A Biol Sci Med Sci* 71: 1661–1666.

Studenski, S., Perera, S., Patel, K., et al. (2011) Gait speed and survival in older adults. *JAMA* 305: 50–58.

Improving Mitochondrial Function

San Millán, I. and Brooks, G.A. (2018) Assessment of metabolic flexibility by means of measuring blood lactate, fat, and carbohydrate oxidation responses to exercise in professional endurance athletes and less-fit individuals. *Sports Med* 48: 467–479.

Achten, J. and Jeukendrup, A.E. (2004) Optimizing fat oxidation through exercise and diet. *Nutrition* 20: 716–727.

de Cabo, R. and Mattson, M.P. (2019) Effects of intermittent fasting on health, aging, and disease. *N Engl J Med* 381: 2541–2551.

Bourguignon, A., Rameau, A., Toullec, G., Romestaing, C. and Roussel, D. (2017) Increased mitochondrial energy efficiency in skeletal muscle after long-term fasting: its relevance to animal performance. *J Exp Biol* 220: 2445–2451.

Miller, B., Hamilton, K., Boushel, R., Williamson, K., Laner, V., Gnaiger, E. and Davis, M. (2017) Mitochondrial respiration in highly aerobic canines in the non-raced state and after a 1600-km sled dog race. *PLoS One* 12: e0174874.

Sies, H., Hollman, P.C., Grune, T., Stahl, W., Biesalski, H.K. and Williamson, G. (2012) Protection by flavanol-rich foods against vascular dysfunction and oxidative damage: 27th Hohenheim Consensus Conference. *Adv Nutr* 3: 217–221.

Aging

van Dam, E., van Leeuwen, L.A.G., Dos Santos, E., James, J., Best, L., Lennicke, C., Vincent, A.J., Marinos, G., Foley, A., Buricova, M., Mokochinski, J.B., Kramer, H.B., Lieb, W., Laudes, M., Franke, A., Kaleta, C. and Cocheme, H.M. (2020) Sugar-induced obesity and insulin resistance are uncoupled from shortened survival in drosophila. *Cell Metab* 31: 710–725 e717.

Roncal-Jimenez, C.A., Ishimoto, T., Lanaspa, M.A., Milagres, T., Hernando, A.A., Jensen, T., Miyazaki, M., Doke, T., Hayasaki, T., Nakagawa, T., Marumaya, S., Long, D.A., Garcia, G.E., Kuwabara, M., Sánchez-Lozada, L.G., Kang, D.H., Johnson, R.J. (2016) Aging-associated renal disease in mice is fructokinase dependent. *Am J Physiol Renal Physiol* 311(4): F722–F730.

Lai, J.Y., Atzmon, G., Melamed, M.L., Hostetter, T.H., Crandall, J.P., Barzilai, N. and Bitzer, M. (2012) Family history of exceptional longevity is associated with lower serum uric acid levels in Ashkenazi Jews. *J Am Geriatr Soc* 60: 745–750.

Supplements and Vitamins

Le, M.T., Lanaspa, M.A., Cicerchi, C.M., et al. (2016) Bioactivity-guided identification of botanical inhibitors of ketohexokinase. *PLoS One* 11: e0157458.

Gutiérrez-Salmeán, G., Meaney, E., Lanaspa, M.A., Cicerchi, C., Johnson, R.J., Dugar, S., Taub, P., Ramírez-Sánchez, I., Villarreal, F., Schreiner, G. and Ceballos, G. (2016) A randomized, placebo-controlled, double-blind study on the effects of (-)-epicatechin on the triglyceride/HDLc ratio and cardiometabolic profile of subjects with hypertriglyceridemia: Unique in vitro effects. *Int J Cardiol* 223: 500–506.

Gomez-Cabrera, M.C., Domenech, E., Romagnoli, M., et al. (2008) Oral administration of vitamin C decreases muscle mitochondrial biogenesis and hampers training-induced adaptations in endurance performance. *American Journal of Clinical Nutrition* 87: 142–149.

García-Arroyo, F.E., Gonzaga-Sánchez, G., Tapia, E., Muñoz-Jiménez, I., Manterola-Romero, L., Osorio-Alonso, H., Arellano-Buendía, A.S., Pedraza-Chaverri, J., Roncal-Jiménez, C.A., Lanaspa, M.A., Johnson, R.J. and Sánchez-Lozada, L.G. (2021) Osthol ameliorates kidney damage and metabolic syndrome induced by a high-fat/high-sugar diet. *Int J Mol Sci* 22: 2431.

A Few Final Words

Benner, S. (2017) Uniting natural history with the molecular sciences. The ultimate multidisciplinarity. *Acc Chem Res* 50: 498–502.

Benner, S.A., Caraco, M.D., Thomson, J.M. and Gaucher, E.A. (2002) Planetary biology—paleontological, geological, and molecular histories of life. *Science* 296: 864–868.

Francey, C., Cros, J., Rosset, R., Crézé, C., Rey, V., Stefanoni, N., Schneiter, P., Tappy, L. and Seyssel, K. (2019) The extra-splanchnic fructose escape after ingestion of a fructose-glucose drink: An exploratory study in healthy humans using a dual fructose isotope method. *Clin Nutr ESPEN* 29: 125–132.

Sherlock Holmes quote from Arthur Conan Doyle. (1890) *The Sign of the Four.* London, Spencer Blackett.

Index

About the Author

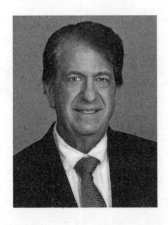

Richard J. Johnson, MD, has been a practicing physician and clinical scientist for over twenty-five years. He is internationally recognized for his seminal work on the role of sugar and its component fructose in obesity and diabetes. His work has also suggested a fundamental role for uric acid (which is generated during fructose metabolism) in metabolic syndrome. Dr. Johnson is a prolific scientist with research that has been funded by the National Institutes of Health since the 1980s. He is a member of the American Society for Clinical Investigation, has published over seven hundred papers and lectured in over forty-five countries, and is a highly cited scientist. He previously authored *The Sugar Fix* with Timothy Gower (Rodale, 2008) and *The Fat Switch* (Mercola.com, 2012). He is currently a professor of medicine at the University of Colorado in Denver. He lives in Aurora, Colorado, with his wife, Olga; his children, Ricky and Tracy; and two miniature goldendoodles, Charlie Brown and Apollo 11.